clinical
examination
essentials

An Introduction to Clinical Skills
(and how to pass your clinical exams)

4TH EDITION

D1354248

clinical examination essentials

An Introduction to Clinical Skills (and how to pass your clinical exams)

4TH EDITION

Nicholas J Talley

MD (NSW), PhD (Syd), MMedSci (Clin Epi)(Newc.), FAHMS, FRACP, FAFPHM, FRCP (Lond), FRCP (Edin), FACP, FACG, AGAF
Laureate Professor of Medicine, Faculty of Health and Medicine, and Pro Vice-Chancellor (Global Research), University of Newcastle, Australia; Senior Staff Specialist, John Hunter Hospital, Newcastle, Australia; Professor of Medicine and Professor of Epidemiology, and Joint Supplemental Consultant Gastroenterology and Health Sciences Research, Mayo Clinic, Rochester, MN, USA

Simon O'Connor

FRACP, DDU, FCSANZ
Cardiologist, The Canberra Hospital;
Clinical Senior Lecturer, Australian National University Medical School, Canberra, Australia

ELSEVIER

ELSEVIER

Elsevier Australia. ACN 001 002 357
(a division of Reed International Books Australia Pty Ltd)
Tower 1, 475 Victoria Avenue, Chatswood, NSW 2067

Notice

This publication has been carefully reviewed and checked to ensure that the content is
as accurate and current as possible at time of publication. We would recommend,
however, that the reader verify any procedures, treatments, drug dosages or legal
content described in this book. Neither the author, the contributors, nor the publisher
assume any liability for injury and/or damage to persons or property arising from any
error in or omission from this publication.

National Library of Australia Cataloguing-in-Publication Data

Talley, Nicholas Joseph, author.

Clinical examination essentials : an introduction to clinical skills (and how to pass your
clinical exams) / Nicholas J Talley & Simon O'Connor.

4th edition.

9780729542289 (paperback)

Includes index.

Physical diagnosis.
Diagnosis.

O'Connor, Simon, author.

616.0754

Content Strategist: Larissa Norrie
Senior Content Development Specialist: Neli Bryant
Project Manager: Devendran Kannan
Edited by Caroline Hunter, Burrumundi Pty Ltd
Proofread by Teresa McIntyre
Design by Toni Darben
Index by Robert Swanson
Typeset by Toppan Best-set Premedia Limited
Printed in China by CTPS

Contents

Foreword

Medicine is a profession that requires an understanding of and an aptitude for science, but also has strong historical and current links to the humanities, and a need to be an excellent and compassionate communicator. This breadth of knowledge and skill is acquired during a long period of training and results in a profession that is always rated by opinion polls as being one of the most respected of all of the professional groups.

Part of the art of medicine is the ability that a competent doctor has to take a concise but comprehensive history, to examine a patient efficiently and proficiently, and to form a differential diagnosis. The education and training needed to develop these skills is complex and requires aptitude and dedication from students and trainees.

A book like this one, which provides a how-to guide to support the next generation of doctors, is an essential toolkit for the doctor in training. Learning clinical skills is the beginning of a fulfilling and wonderful career as a medical professional. These days, being a doctor can be tough, as the increasing needs of patients with multiple problems become more difficult to deal with and the rapid expansion of medical knowledge is more difficult to keep up with. Becoming as proficient as possible in the practice of your clinical skills will help to make you as good a doctor as it is possible to be.

Professor Jane Dacre
BSc, MBBS, MD, FRCP (Lond), FRCP (Edin), FRCPS (Glas), FHEA
President, Royal College of Physicians of London, UK;
Professor of Medical Education, UCL, London, UK;
Consultant physician and rheumatologist,
Whittington Hospital, London, UK

Preface

It is much simpler to buy books than to read them and easier to read them than to absorb their contents.

Sir William Osler (1849–1919)

This fourth edition of *clinical examination essentials* has been written to assist medical students to begin their clinical journey and attain competence in history taking and physical examination. We have also included material that more experienced medical students will want to refer to again and again as they practise their clinical skills and prepare for their barrier clinical examinations.

Clinical examinations often seem an artificial way to test students' knowledge. Taking a history from or performing an examination of a patient while being watched by examiners is very challenging and stressful. However, the more the techniques of history taking and examination are practised, the less difficult it becomes to perform them under observation—they become second nature. This, we believe, is the main point of clinical exams: they force you to spend considerable time seeing patients so that you can practise and become familiar with these essential aspects of medical practice. On the journey towards clinical competence, history taking and physical examination are essential skills for all doctors.

This book sets out approaches to history taking and examination techniques for those students learning these skills for the first time as well as for those revising before their clinical exams. The book is meant to be a guide and it is important that you develop your own approach. We emphasise in this book the need to practise and observe: medicine is not learned from the computer or phone screen, or from the written page, but by meeting and examining real people who deserve our deep respect and who trust us to put their best interests before our own, as we must. Examiners can soon tell which students have learned to think and act like a doctor.

We have included examination hint boxes throughout the text. These emphasise particular points likely to be useful during the OSCEs (objective structured clinical examinations) and other examinations. The book is not a substitute for hard work on the wards: to become competent, you must talk to and examine as many patients as possible during your clinical rotations. You will learn most from your interactions with patients. There is no single correct way to assess patients on the wards or during clinical exams but there are obvious mistakes to avoid and techniques that work, as we point out in the pages that follow.

Advances in technology are stunning, but even today in about 80% of cases the diagnosis of a medical condition is made, or strongly suspected, on the basis of the history and examination. Accurate diagnosis is so important because treatment usually flows from it; an incorrectly taken history that leads to a wrong diagnosis can (and does) lead to harm. Tests ordered for the wrong reasons, because the patient's story has not been properly obtained, are often useless—or worse, dangerous.

In this edition we have included clinical photographs that have largely replaced line drawings in order to communicate more clearly the key information and illustrate key physical signs. Anatomical information, including surface anatomy, is included because anatomy is the foundation of correct physical examination—you must know what is normal and what structures underlie each part of the body to appreciate abnormalities.

There are new jokes (some understated, some not so subtle) because we firmly believe that learning should be fun and medicine a pleasure to master. As with all our books, this book has undergone peer review to ensure that the material is relevant and contemporary. We welcome feedback and suggestions to aid learning. Please contact us via the publisher if you have any suggestions or ideas for the next edition.

We hope you will be inspired to master clinical skills by using this book. Our companion and larger textbook, *Clinical Examination: A Systematic Guide to Physical Diagnosis*, provides greater detail for more senior students and graduates. The journey here is as important as the end result, so please enjoy it. We wish you every success!

Nicholas J Talley & Simon O'Connor
Newcastle and Canberra, September 2015

Reviewers

We are very grateful for the thoughtful and professional reviews received that have helped us to further strengthen each edition. We are convinced that peer review is essential not just to judge original research findings but also to advance the quality of medical education, including the accuracy and excellence of textbooks. We extend our appreciation to the following reviewers for their comments and insights into the fourth edition:

Gerry Corrigan BA, DipEd, PhD, MACE
Associate Professor of Medical Education, ANU Medical School, Australian National University, Canberra, ACT, Australia

Michael Dodson MBBS, BSc, BMedSci, MPH, MHM, PhD
Medical Director, Blackmores Ltd; Adjunct Associate Professor, University of Western Sydney, New South Wales, Australia

Robert Paul Dowsett BMBS, DipCE, FACEM
Senior Lecturer, Department of Medical Education, Faculty of Medicine, Dentistry and Health Sciences, The University of Melbourne, Victoria, Australia

Karen D'Souza MBBS (Hons)
Senior Lecturer in Medical Education (Coordinator of Clinical Skills, Curriculum and Assessment Theme), School of Medicine, Deakin University, Victoria, Australia

Balakrishnan Kichu Nair AM, MBBS, MD, FRACP, FRCPE, FRCPG, FRCPI, FANZSGM

Professor of Medicine & Associate Dean, School of Medicine, University of Newcastle; Adjunct Professor, University of New England; Director, Centre for Medical Professional Development, HNE Health, Newcastle, New South Wales, Australia

Ian Symonds MD, MMedSci, FRCOG, FRANZCOG

Professor of Obstetrics & Gynaecology, University of Newcastle, New South Wales, Australia

Jonathan Williamson MBBS, PhD, FRACP

Staff Specialist, Respiratory and Sleep Physician, Liverpool Hospital; VMO, Macquarie University Hospital, New South Wales, Australia

Nicola Wood BMed, BMedSci (Honours)

Junior Medical Officer, Hunter New England Health Network, New South Wales, Australia

Taking the history

*In taking histories, follow each line of thought; ask
no leading questions; never suggest. Give the
patient's own words in the complaint.*
  *Never ask a new patient a question without a
notebook and pencil in hand.*

Sir William Osler (1849–1919)

This is arguably the most important chapter that you'll read in
medical school. Even in the twenty-first century, with all the
rapid and exciting advances in biology and computing, excellent
history taking remains absolutely central to best practice in
medicine. Practising medicine remains an art and a science:
competence comes only with experience. Here you will begin to
learn how to acquire the necessary skills, which with practice
(and you must practise) should become second nature.

The history: rationale

The patient must be your primary concern. As a doctor (or
medical student), you have a fundamental duty to understand
your patients' stories, including the background context. To help
and to heal, you need to learn what your patients have experienced and what they feel. Long case examinations and history
taking OSCEs test these skills, sometimes with real patients and
sometimes with trained actor-patients.

T&O'C examination hint box

Medical student alert
To be rated excellent on ward rounds in your clinical rotations (and help out busy resident doctors who may have had to take short cuts):
- know each patient's complete history, examination and test results so that you can contribute to the discussions (and upstage any resident doctors who have taken short cuts)
- offer to admit patients and write in the notes
- help to position patients or adjust the bed and ensure that patients are always comfortable[1]
- do a pre-ward round—talk to patients, read their notes and look up management of their problems (aim to know more than the resident doctors)
- take seriously what the nurses tell you—they are often very experienced and knowledgeable about patients and can help steer you away from making major errors as a recent graduate
- turn off or silence your mobile phone during the rounds.

Make up to the resident doctor for showing him or her up during rounds by:[2]
- offering to see new patients first and helping with the admission notes (taking the history and doing the examination)
- offering to take blood, insert cannulas etc.

- While every story is unique, in most cases doctors can deduce a reasonable diagnosis by listening carefully and asking the right questions.
- By narrowing the differential diagnosis (a list of the possible diagnoses suggested by a set of symptoms or signs), appropriate testing and therapy can be ordered.

Remember:
- *Symptoms* are subjective feelings perceptible to the patient, while *signs* are changes that can be demonstrated objectively. For example, diarrhoea is a symptom and if you take the time to look at the stool yourself, it can also be a sign.
- In clinical practice the history is used to help direct the physical examination to the appropriate part of the body.

---

1 Focus on patient privacy and comfort: this will be appreciated and will enhance the clinical encounter.
2 Offering to wash his or her car or bicycle might be a bit obvious.

For example, in a patient presenting with a cough the respiratory and cardiovascular systems will need to be examined.

- Even if the possible diagnoses are not clear after the history has been taken, it will usually be obvious which body region or system is affected. This will enable you to direct the examination and diagnostic tests appropriately.

Unless patients are extremely ill, the taking of a careful medical history should precede both examination and treatment. Taking the history and examining the patient are also, of course, the least expensive ways of making a diagnosis. *A good history will usually take you 80% of the way to making the right diagnosis.*

Bedside manner

The word 'clinical' is derived from the Greek word *klīnikós*, meaning 'of or pertaining to a bed' (*Oxford English Dictionary*, 2nd edn). The term 'bedside manner' describes the clinician's approach to the patient.

- Doctors hold a privileged position because they are told confidential information about patients and their families. As a professional, you must act with honesty and integrity and treat patients as individuals with respect and dignity.
- Using a professional manner will make history taking and physical examination enjoyable and rewarding for both you and the patient.
- Excellence in bedside manner is learnt by observing the methods (both successful and unsuccessful) of senior colleagues.
- After the examination, offer an explanation to the patient of the expected diagnosis and the prognosis (the likely outcome of the illness), but this should not extend beyond what the patient has already been told by more senior medical staff. It may, however, be an opportunity to answer the patient's questions and offer explanations.
- This may also be the time to discuss investigations and treatment (if you can think of any).
- Remember that the clinician's recommendations are just that—it should be clear to patients that they can freely accept or reject these recommendations (except in the most unusual circumstances).

Obtaining the history

The medical interview deals not only with the patient's bodily problems but also with any psychosocial aspects of the patient's illness: the mind and body are not separate entities. Points to remember:

- The information you are told is confidential and the medical records form a legal document.
- Make your patient feel safe (e.g. maximise privacy, introduce yourself, maintain appropriate eye contact) and comfortable (e.g. check that the patient is feeling physically comfortable).
- Make a conscious effort to listen to the patient and to establish rapport (active listening).
- You should be dressed modestly and smartly to gain the patient's confidence.
- Write rough notes while questioning the patient. You can make a more detailed record at the end of the history taking and examination (this is often dictated or entered into a computer record).
- The record should be a *sequential*, accurate account of the development and course of the patient's illness or illnesses (even if this is not the order in which the questions were asked).
- A systematic approach to history taking and recording is the most reliable way to avoid missing crucial information (see Box 1.1).
- The record must make it clear whether the patient's problem is one of **diagnosis** (i.e. what is wrong) or **management** (i.e. what tests and treatment are necessary), or **both**.

PRINCIPLES OF PATIENT-CENTRED HISTORY TAKING

- Sit down beside the patient to be as close to their eye level as possible (don't let the computer get in the way), and ensure that you give the impression that the interview will be unhurried (see Fig 1.1).
- Establish a good relationship, maximising privacy and eye contact.
- Use open questions.

> **Box 1.1**
> **History-taking sequence**
>
> **Presenting (principal) symptom (PS)**
> A list of the main complaint(s) in the patient's own words
>
> **History of presenting illness (HPI)**
> Details of current symptoms or complaints
> Details of previous similar episodes
> Current and recent treatment (all drugs: doses, duration, indication)
> Extent of functional disability
>
> **Past history (PH)**
> Past illnesses
> Past surgical operations (dates and indications)
> Past treatments (drugs, transfusions)
> Drug allergies
> Health maintenance (disease prevention)
> Menstrual and reproductive history for women
>
> **Social history (SH)**
> Occupation, education, place of birth
> Marital status, social support, living conditions
> Smoking history and alcohol use
> Use of analgesics
> Overseas travel (where and when)
> Sexual and drug abuse history (if relevant)
>
> **Family history (FH)**
> Diseases in first-degree relatives
>
> **Systems review (SR)**
> Incorporate into the sections above

- Interview in a logical manner.
- Listen carefully and note non-verbal clues.
- Interrupt appropriately (focusing on encouraging the patient to tell the full story in his or her own words first).
- Correctly interpret the information obtained.

INTRODUCTORY QUESTIONS

Introduce yourself to the patient. It is important to address the patient respectfully and to use his or her name and title. It is usually sufficient to introduce yourself to the patient as a student doctor.

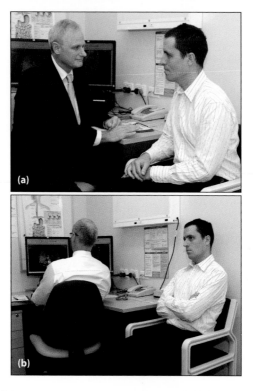

Figure 1.1 Correct **(a)** and incorrect **(b)** interviewing position.

Find out the patient's major complaint or complaints. It is best to attempt a conversational approach and ask 'What has been the trouble or problem recently?' or 'When did these problems begin?' If the patient has already been interviewed by the resident, the registrar, the consultant and three medical students, it may be necessary to apologise and explain the importance of you hearing about the problem in the patient's own words.

- Allow the patient to tell the whole story if possible, then ask questions to fill in the gaps.
- Use appropriate (but not exaggerated) reassuring gestures.
- If the patient stops giving the history spontaneously, it can be helpful to provide a short summary of what has already been said and then encourage the patient to continue.

- Learn to listen with an open mind and resist the temptation to leap to specific questions before the patient has had a chance to describe all the symptoms in his or her own words. However, some direction may be necessary to keep a talkative patient on track.
- Avoid using pseudo-medical terms and, if the patient uses them, find out exactly what the patient means, because misinterpretation of medical terms is common.

While the patient is describing the symptoms, make observations to help you draw inferences about the patient's personality. For example, note:

- the patient's dress and facial expressions (e.g. the amount of distress while describing personal matters)
- any signs of anxiety or restlessness and mannerisms (remember, the patient may notice signs of restlessness or anxiety in you if lunchtime is approaching).

T&O'C examination hint box

The experienced clinician tries to deal with each of the patient's major symptoms in turn. This may mean interrupting the patient if he or she is keen to move onto another symptom before you have asked all the questions you need to about the previous symptom. This must always be done politely. For example, you could say, 'I'd just like to finish asking you about your blackouts before we talk about your tiredness.'

THE PRESENTING (PRINCIPAL OR CHIEF) SYMPTOM (OR COMPLAINT) (PS)

The presenting (principal or chief) symptom is the symptom or problem that has led the patient to come for help. It must be remembered that the patient's and the doctor's ideas of what constitutes a serious problem may differ.

CURRENT SYMPTOMS AND HISTORY OF THE PRESENTING ILLNESS (HPI)

Quite a lot of detail about the course and nature of *all* of the patient's symptoms is required. The history of the presenting illness should be written so that the events are placed in chronological order or, if numerous systems are affected, they are in chronological order for each system. Certain information should routinely be sought for each symptom if this isn't volunteered by the patient. The mnemonic SOCRATES summarises the questions that should be asked about each symptom:

- **S**ite
- **O**nset
- **C**haracter and severity
- **R**adiation
- **A**ggravating and relieving factors
- **T**iming
- **E**xacerbating factors and associated symptoms
- **S**ocial effects of the symptoms or illness.

Site

- Ask where the symptom is exactly and whether it is localised or diffuse. Ask the patient to point to the actual site, if localised.

Onset

- Find out when the symptom first began and try to date this as accurately as possible.
- A patient asked 'How long has this pain been present?' will not uncommonly say, 'For a long time, doctor'. It is necessary then to ask 'Do you mean a few hours or many weeks?' Although you should not suggest answers to the patient, giving a few possible alternatives may speed up the process.
- The time of the day may be relevant. For example, the joint pain and stiffness of rheumatoid arthritis are worst on waking, while the pain of osteoarthritis becomes worse during the day.

Character and severity

- Ask the patient to clarify what he or she means by the symptom. For example, if the patient complains of dizziness, does this mean the room spins around (vertigo) or is it more a feeling of light-headedness?
- It may be necessary to suggest some alternative descriptions. For example, a patient may find chest discomfort difficult to describe. It is thus reasonable to ask whether the feeling is tight, heavy, sharp or stabbing. (It is interesting to note that patients who have been stabbed do not usually describe the pain as stabbing.)

- Symptom severity is subjective. The best way to assess severity is to ask the patient whether the symptom interferes with normal activities or sleep.
- It may be useful to ask the patient to grade pain as a number between 0 and 10, where 10 represents the most severe pain the patient has ever experienced and 0 represents no pain. Alternatively, you can ask whether pain, or another symptom, is mild, moderate, severe or very severe.

Radiation

- Ask whether the symptom, if localised, radiates (travels elsewhere, especially pain). The pattern of radiation is very suggestive of certain abnormalities—for example, the distribution of pain and paraesthesias (pins and needles) in the territory of the median nerve of the hand in carpal tunnel syndrome or the radiation of pain through to the back in pancreatitis.
- Symptoms such as cough, dyspnoea (shortness of breath), change in weight or dizziness are not localised.

Aggravating and relieving factors

- Ask whether anything makes the symptom worse or better. For example, lying flat may make the dyspnoea of heart failure worse but not that of chronic obstructive pulmonary disease (sometimes called chronic bronchitis or emphysema). Exercise brings on chest pain from angina that is relieved by rest.

Timing

- Find out whether the symptom came on rapidly, gradually or instantaneously. Certain symptoms are typically very sudden in onset (like turning on a light)— for example, the onset of a fast heartbeat in supraventricular tachycardia.
- Ask whether the symptom is present continuously or intermittently.
- Find out whether the symptom is becoming worse or better and, if so, when the change occurred. Some symptoms are at their very worst at the moment of onset (e.g. the pain of an aortic tear called a dissection). Find out what the patient was doing at the time the symptom began.

Exacerbating factors and associated symptoms

- Attempt to uncover in a systematic way symptoms that might be expected to be associated with a particular disease or risk factors that make a disease more likely. For example, a strong family history of carcinoma of the colon makes rectal bleeding a more sinister symptom.
- For a patient who presents with cardiac symptoms, the major risk factors for coronary artery disease (e.g. smoking and family history) must be assessed in detail.

Social effects of the symptoms or illness

- Any serious or chronic illness may cause severe financial or social problems that should be explored and documented. These problems need to be taken into account when planning the best treatment for a patient.

Current treatment

- Ask the patient whether he or she is currently taking any tablets or medicines or using skin patches. Attempt to find out the names and doses of each, and the reason for taking the medicine.
- Always ask whether a woman is taking the contraceptive pill because it is not considered a medicine or tablet by many who take it.
- Remember, patients may think that non-prescription drugs are not relevant; ask about them specifically.
- Also ask about alternative treatments including vitamin or mineral supplements.
- Medicines may give a clue to unrecognised medical problems (e.g. a patient who takes glucosamine is likely to have arthritis).

PAST HISTORY (PH)

Establish systematically aspects of the patient's past history that have not yet emerged.

Past illnesses and surgical operations

- Ask the patient whether he or she has had any serious illnesses, operations or admissions to hospital. If so, establish at what age these occurred, the indications for any operations and any serious illnesses in childhood that interfered with school.

- Patients are not always correct about their previous diagnoses. Questions about how a diagnosis was made may be required to help clarify things.
- A history of multiple accidents or serious illnesses may suggest an underlying problem. For example, alcohol or drug abuse may be the cause of repeated motor accidents or head injuries. Elderly patients may have multiple falls because of neurological or bone disease.

Past treatments

- Some medications or treatments that a patient has had in the past may remain relevant, including:
  - corticosteroids
  - oral contraceptives
  - antihypertensive agents
  - blood transfusions
  - chemotherapy or radiotherapy for malignancy.

Drug allergies

- Note any adverse reactions that have occurred in the past.
- Ask what any allergic reaction actually involved. Often, patients may confuse an allergy with the side effects of a drug (e.g. nausea after narcotic administration is a side effect not an allergy), but these reactions should still be documented.

Health maintenance

- Ask about immunisation status and recent vaccinations.
- Establish details about past screening tests, such as the Papanicolaou (Pap) smear, mammography, chest X-rays, faecal occult blood testing or colonoscopy.

Menstrual and reproductive history

- This information is particularly relevant for a woman with abdominal pain, a suspected endocrine disease or genitourinary symptoms.
- Ask at what age menstruation began, whether the periods have a regular cycle and whether menopause has occurred.
- Note the date of the last menstrual period.

- Ask a woman in the childbearing years if there is a possibility that she might be pregnant, as this may preclude the use of certain investigations (e.g. those involving X-rays) and drugs.
- The reproductive history can be written in shorthand as *gravida*, *para*, X-X-X-X, where:
    - gravida is the total number of pregnancies (including a current one)
    - para is the number of deliveries after 20 weeks of pregnancy
    - X-X-X-X refers to the number of full-term infants, the number of pre-term infants, the number of abortions and the number of living children, respectively.

SOCIAL HISTORY (SH)

The social history encompasses the patient's economic, social, domestic and industrial situation. Social factors influence disease outcomes and/or may contribute to disease development.

Occupation, education and place of birth

- Ask the patient about his or her present occupation and what he or she does at work. Note particularly:
    - any work exposure to dusts, chemicals or disease—for example, mine workers may have the disease silicosis, even if they worked in the mines many years ago
    - whether the patient has a sedentary or a physically active job, as this will have implications for return to work after an illness.
- Also ask about hobbies, which may be informative (e.g. bird fanciers lung disease).
- Ask about the patient's:
    - level of education
    - place of birth and residence
    - ethnic background (this predisposes patients to some diseases, such as thalassaemia and sickle cell anaemia).

Marital status, social support and living conditions

- Ask who lives at home with the patient, and about the patient's marital status or other living arrangements and the home environment. Enquire whether there is anyone to help with convalescence.

- Is the patient's partner male or female?
- Find out about the health of the patient's spouse or partner and any children.

Social habits

- This is the time when possibly awkward questions about the patient's social habits should be asked. It is always best to sound matter-of-fact when asking these questions.

Smoking

- A patient may claim to be a non-smoker if he or she stopped smoking that morning. Therefore, you must ask:
  - whether the patient has ever smoked
  - if so, how many cigarettes (or cigars or pipes) were smoked a day and for how many years—this is often recorded in packet-years, with a standard packet of cigarettes considered to be 20, so 20 cigarettes a day for a year = 1 packet-year and 30 cigarettes a day for 20 years = 30 packet-years
  - about e-cigarette use.
- Cigarette smoking is a risk factor for vascular disease, chronic lung disease and several cancers. It may also damage a fetus. The risks of e-cigarettes are uncertain.

Alcohol

- Ask whether the patient drinks alcohol. It is useful to ask:
  - what the patient usually drinks (e.g. beer or wine)
  - how many glasses the patient drinks per day. It can be useful to 'adjust up' the patient's estimate (e.g. 'So you drink about 10 beers a day; do you drink any spirits?'), giving the patient the chance to modify the original claim without embarrassment.
- One standard drink is one glass of wine, one glass of standard-strength beer or one nip of spirit.
- Guidelines for safe alcohol drinking vary. If a patient drinks more than 2 standard drinks daily or more than 4 standard drinks on a single day, he or she may be at risk. Women and older patients (≥65 years) generally should not drink more than 7 standard drinks per week. At least

2 alcohol-free days per week is recommended for men and women.

- To screen for unhealthy drinking, ask 'How many times in the past year have you had 5 (for men)/4 (for women) or more drinks in a day?' If the answer is 'I don't remember', suspect alcohol abuse and try to probe for more detail.

Analgesics

- If the patient has not already volunteered information about the use of analgesics, ask about these medicines.
- Aspirin and other non-steroidal anti-inflammatory drugs (NSAIDs), but not paracetamol (acetaminophen), can cause:
  - peptic ulcers
  - gastrointestinal bleeding (COX-2 selective inhibitors much less than traditional NSAIDs)
  - asthma
  - kidney disease.
- Most NSAIDs (but not aspirin) increase the risk of myocardial infarction.
- Opioids are commonly prescribed for pain and may cause constipation.

Overseas travel

- If an infectious disease is a possibility, ask about:
  - recent overseas travel and destinations visited
  - how the patient lived when away
  - prophylaxis given to protect against diseases such as malaria
  - vaccination against hepatitis (A and B), rabies, typhoid etc.
- People who were born or have lived for long periods overseas may acquire diseases such as tuberculosis.
- Note that the migrant parents of children born in Australia or New Zealand often do not realise their children need vaccination when they travel to their home country.

SEXUAL AND DRUG ABUSE HISTORY

Approaching this topic is never easy for the doctor or the patient. You may wish to preface these questions with a statement such as: 'I need to ask you some personal questions because they may be relevant to your current state of health.' It is not your role to make judgements about a person's life.

The patient's sexual history may be relevant if HIV (human immunodeficiency virus) is suspected or if there is a history of:

- urethral discharge
- dysuria (burning or pain on urination)
- vaginal discharge
- a genital ulcer or rash
- pain on intercourse
- anorectal symptoms.

If a sexually transmitted infection may be the problem, a detailed sexual history will be required. Determine:

- the date of last intercourse
- the number of contacts
- any same-sex partners
- contacts with sex workers.

The type of sexual practice may also be important—for example:

- oro-anal contact may predispose to colonic infection
- peri-rectal contact may predispose to hepatitis B or C or HIV infection
- inserting objects into the rectum may cause trauma that is otherwise difficult to explain.

Marijuana has been legalised in a number of countries and is commonly used as a medicine as well as recreationally. Ask about this and other drugs, including cocaine.

The use of intravenous drugs has many implications for the patient's health. If the patient uses such drugs, ask whether an attempt is made to avoid the sharing of needles. This may protect against the injection of viruses but not against bacterial infection from the use of impure substances.

T&O'C examination hint box

There is controversy concerning the taking of a detailed sexual history from a patient you have met for the first time in a long case examination. It may be reasonable to tell the examiner that you would defer this questioning until you know the patient better, unless it is directly relevant (e.g. a patient with HIV).

FAMILY HISTORY (FH)

Many diseases run in families. It is worth asking specifically about a family history of heart disease, stroke, diabetes, alcoholism or bleeding tendencies—for example:

- ischaemic heart disease in parents who developed this at a young age is a major risk factor for ischaemic heart disease in their offspring
- various malignancies, such as breast and colon carcinoma, are more common in certain families
- some diseases are directly inherited (e.g. haemophilia); ask whether similar illnesses have occurred in family members.

SYSTEMS REVIEW (SR)

As well as detailed questioning about the system likely to be diseased, it is essential to ask about important symptoms and disorders in other systems, otherwise important diseases may be missed. The extent of this review depends on the presenting problem and circumstances: an 18-year-old needing sutures removed will clearly require fewer questions than a 75-year-old with multiple medical problems. Ask some general questions first, then begin the questioning for each system with a general question about any history of heart or lung trouble and so on (see Box 1.2). Decide how detailed the questioning needs to be: it is not usually necessary to ask all of the questions listed in Box 1.2.

Concluding the interview

- Always ask, 'Is anything else troubling you?' Sometimes, you'll be amazed by the new information gleaned.
- Remember that as a student you may have more time—and in an examination, more incentive—than anyone else to take a detailed history and it is possible that you will uncover new information. Advise the patient that it is important to add this information to the documented history and ensure that you advise the registrar or consultant.
- Ask whether the patient has any questions, and whether any close relatives or friends should be involved in subsequent discussions about your recommendations.
- Explain the next steps after making your recommendations.
- If your recommendations are repeatedly rejected by your patients, you have probably made a poor attempt at explaining them. Consider a career as a medical administrator.

Box 1.2
The systems review

❗ denotes symptoms for the possible diagnosis of an urgent or dangerous problem (red flag symptom)

General questions
❗ • Have you noticed shivering or sweating at night or have you had a high temperature?
❗ • Have you unintentionally lost weight recently?
   • Have there been changes in your appetite?
   • Have there been changes in your pattern of sleep?
   • Have you felt that your mood has changed?

Cardiovascular system
❗ • Have you had any pain or pressure in your chest? If so, does this occur during exertion? (Angina)
   • Are you short of breath on exertion? (Dyspnoea) If so, how much exertion is necessary? How many flights of stairs can you climb before you start to become short of breath?
❗ • Have you ever been woken at night by severe shortness of breath? (Paroxysmal nocturnal dyspnoea)
   • Can you lie flat without feeling breathless? (Orthopnoea)
   • Have you had swelling of your ankles? (Peripheral oedema) Or varicose veins?
   • Have you noticed your heart racing or beating irregularly?
   • Do you have pain in your calves on walking? (Claudication)
   • Do you have cold or blue hands or feet? (Peripheral cyanosis)
   • Have you had rheumatic fever, a heart attack or high blood pressure?
   • Also ask about specific cardiovascular risk factors:
     – Has your cholesterol level been checked recently? If so, has it been treated or left untreated?
     – Have you been diagnosed with diabetes mellitus? If so, for how long?
     – Do you smoke? If so, for how long, how many?
     – Do you have a family history of cardiovascular disease? If so, who and at what age?

Respiratory system
❗ • Are you short of breath at rest?
   • Have you had any cough?
   • Do you cough up anything? (Productive cough)
❗ • Have you coughed up blood? (Haemoptysis, carcinoma of the lung)
   • Do you snore loudly or fall asleep during the day unexpectedly? (Possible obstructive sleep apnoea)

continued

Box 1.2
The systems review *continued*

- Do you ever have wheezing when you are short of breath? (Bronchospasm)
- Do you have night sweats?
- Have you had pneumonia or tuberculosis?
- Have you had a recent chest X-ray?

Gastrointestinal system
- Have you had a sore tongue or mouth ulcers?
- Are you troubled by indigestion? If so, what do you mean by indigestion?
! • Have you had any difficulty swallowing? (Dysphagia: oesophageal malignancy)
- Has your appetite or weight changed? If so, how has it changed?
- Have you had episodes of burning discomfort in the chest that rises up towards the neck? (Heartburn)
- Have you been taking antacids or over-the-counter indigestion medicines?
- Have you been taking laxatives or tablets for diarrhoea?
- Have you had pain or discomfort in your belly (tummy)?
- Have you had any bloating or visible swelling of your belly?
- Has your bowel habit changed recently?
- How many bowel motions do you usually pass per day?
- Have you lost control of your bowels or had accidents? (Faecal incontinence)
- Have you seen blood in your motions or on wiping? (Haematochezia)
! • Have you vomited blood or had black bowel motions? (Melaena)
- Do you take laxatives or use enemas?
- Have your eyes or skin ever been yellow? (Jaundice)
- Have you noticed dark urine and pale stools?
- Have you had hepatitis, peptic ulceration, colitis or bowel cancer?
- Tell me about your diet recently.

Genitourinary system and sexual health
- Do you have burning or pain on passing urine? (Dysuria)
- Is your urine stream as good as it used to be?
- Is there a delay before you start to pass urine? (Hesitancy)
- Is there dribbling at the end when you pass urine?
- Do you have to get up at night to pass urine? (Nocturia)
- Are you passing larger or smaller amounts of urine?
- Have you noticed leaking of urine? (Incontinence)
- Has your urine colour changed? Is your urine dark?

Box 1.2
The systems review   *continued*

- Have you seen blood in your urine? (Haematuria)
- Have you had a urinary tract infection or kidney stones?
- Do you have any problems with your sex life?
- Have you noticed any rashes or lumps on your genitals?
- Have you had a sexually transmitted infection?
- Do you have difficulty maintaining an erection?
- Have you had penile discharge or skin lesions?
- Have you ever felt lumps in your testes?
- Are your periods regular? At what age did you begin to menstruate (menarche)?
- Do you have excessive pain (dysmenorrhoea) or bleeding (menorrhagia) with your periods?
- Do you have bleeding after sex?
- Have you had any miscarriages?
- Have you had high blood pressure or diabetes in pregnancy?

Breasts (women)
- Have you had any bleeding or discharge from your breasts?
- ! Have you felt any lumps in or around your breasts?
- Have you had a recent mammogram, ultrasound or breast examination?

Haematological system
- Do you bruise easily?
- Have you had bleeding from your gums? (Bleeding disorder or leukaemia)
- Have you had fevers, or shivers and shakes (rigors)?
- Do you have difficulty stopping a small cut from bleeding?
- Have you noticed any lumps under your arms, or in your neck or groin? (Lymphadenopathy)
- Have you had blood clots in your legs (venous thrombosis) or lungs (pulmonary embolism)?
- Have you had anaemia?

Musculoskeletal system
- Do you have painful or swollen joints? If so, what joints are affected?
- Do you suffer from morning stiffness? If so, how long does it last?
- Are your joints ever hot, red or swollen?
- Have you had frequent muscle pains or cramps?
- Have you had a skin rash recently?
- Do you have any back or neck pain?
- Have your eyes been dry or red?
- Is your mouth often dry? (Sjögren's syndrome)

continued

Box 1.2
The systems review *continued*

- Have you been diagnosed as having rheumatoid arthritis or gout?
- Do your fingers ever become painful and go white, then blue, then red in the cold? (Raynaud's phenomenon)
- How much do your joint problems interfere with normal activities?

Endocrine system
- Have you noticed any swelling in your neck? (Goitre)
- Do your hands tremble (tremor)?
- Do you prefer hot or cold weather?
- Have you had a thyroid problem or diabetes?
- Have you noticed increased sweating?
- Have you been troubled by fatigue?
- Have you noticed any change in your appearance, hair, skin or voice?
- Have you noticed a change in your hat, glove or shoe size? (Acromegaly)
! • Have you been unusually thirsty lately? (Uncontrolled diabetes)
- Have you been passing large amounts of urine? (Polyuria)

Neurological system
- Do you get headaches?
- Have you had memory problems or trouble concentrating?
! • Have you had fainting episodes, fits or blackouts?
- Do you have double vision (diplopia) or other trouble seeing or hearing?
- Are you dizzy? Does the world seem to turn around? (Vertigo)
- Have you had weakness, numbness or clumsiness in your arms or legs, or trouble with your balance or walking?
! • Have you had a stroke or serious head injury?
- Have you had difficulty sleeping?
- Do you feel sad or depressed or have problems with your nerves?
! • Have you ever considered suicide?

Skin
- Have you had itching (pruritus) or a rash?
- Have you had similar rashes in the past?
- When did the problem start?
- Has the rash changed or become more widespread over time?
- Have you had any recent illnesses or travelled anywhere?
- Have you had asthma or allergic rhinitis? (Atopy)
- What work do you do? (Contact dermatitis)
- Have you noticed moles that have changed?
- Has there been a change in your hair or nails?
- Have you had lumps or frequent infections in your skin?

T&O'C examination hint box

During the interview, ask the patient 'Is there anything else?' whenever a natural break in the history taking occurs.

T&O'C examination essentials

Taking a better history

Listen to the patient. He is telling you the diagnosis.

Sir William Osler (1849–1919)

1. Allow the patient to tell the story in his or her own words. Establish rapport and listen with enthusiasm. Ask specific questions to fill in the gaps, then ask the patient whether there is anything else he or she would like to discuss.
2. Make sure the patient does not have the impression that the interview is being hurried (except in an emergency).
3. Concentrate on the history of the presenting illness. This must be documented sequentially and in the greatest detail.
4. Incorporate the relevant symptoms obtained in the systems review in the history of the presenting illness.
5. Remember that the past history, social history and family history are often highly relevant to the presenting illness.
6. Explore psychological matters where they may be relevant.
7. Don't accept one-line answers and don't be content with facts that seem contradictory or chronologically obscure; trust, but always verify.
8. Use systematic questions about potential risk factors for various diseases to assist in establishing the diagnosis (e.g. smoking and coronary artery disease).
9. Remember that constant practice is needed to become a proficient history taker.
10. A good interview has genuine therapeutic value.
11. The best doctors take and document great histories!

Advanced
history taking

*Acquire the art of detachment, the virtue of method,
and the quality of thoroughness, but above all the
grace of humility.*

*A patient with a written list of symptoms—
neurasthenia.*[1]

Sir William Osler (1849–1919)

To conduct a successful patient-centred interview, you must
develop rapport and trust. Certain aspects of history taking go
beyond routine questioning about symptoms. This part of the art
has to be learned by taking a lot of histories: practice is absolutely
essential. With time you will gain confidence in dealing with
patients whose psychiatric, cultural or medical situation makes
standard questioning difficult or impossible.

History taking for the maintenance
of good health

The first interview with a patient is an opportunity to make an
assessment of the known risk factors for a number of important

---

1 Neurasthenia refers to 'nervous exhaustion' and includes symptoms from anxiety and
depression to multiple unexplained bodily complaints such as fatigue, backache and
headache. It is now termed somatic symptom disorder.

Box 2.1
Useful routine questions to help patients to maintain good health

Ask patients about the following
- Smoking habits and cholesterol level
- Diet and consumption of alcohol
- Level of exercise
- Current weight, and any recent change in weight
- Practices related to sexual health
- Vaccinations (for adults over 18 years of age; see also www.cdc.gov/vaccines/schedules/index.html and www.immunise.health.gov.au/internet/immunise/publishing.nsf/Content/nips-ctn):
  - *Haemophilus influenzae* type b
  - hepatitis A and B
  - human papillomavirus (females ≤26 years only)
  - influenza (annually, if at increased risk)
  - measles, mumps, rubella
  - meningococcal
  - pneumococcal
  - tetanus, diphtheria, pertussis (every 10 years)
  - varicella zoster (60 years and older)
- Screening for breast cancer and ovarian cancer (family history, or age 50 years plus)
- Screening for colon cancer (age 50 years plus, or family history of colon cancer or personal history of inflammatory bowel disease)
- Family history of other inherited diseases (may be an indication for screening tests, e.g. hypertrophic cardiomyopathy)
- Family history of sudden death

medical conditions (see Box 2.1). Even when a patient has come about an unconnected problem, there is often the opportunity for a quick review of these factors. Constant matter-of-fact reminders about these things can make a great deal of difference to the way people protect themselves from ill-health.

- Most people have some understanding of the dangers associated with smoking, excessive alcohol consumption and obesity. People have more varied views on what constitutes a healthy diet and exercise regimen, and many are ignorant of what constitutes risky sexual activity.
- Part of the thorough assessment of a patient includes obtaining and conveying some idea of what measures may help the patient to maintain good health. This includes a

Tips for a successful patient-centred consultation
- Make the patient feel welcome and comfortable. Make the patient the centre of your universe for this period.
- Welcome the patient's partner or relatives to attend the consultation, but only if the patient wants them to attend (and not too many at once).
- Actively listen and find out about the patient as a person.
- Take all of the patient's problems seriously.
- Be polite and never be judgemental.
- Avoid excitability; speak clearly and not too fast.
- Take no short cuts—where possible, take as long as is needed: all relevant questions need to be asked.
- Show you care by your manner and responses.
- Look professional: be well groomed and tidy.
- Be professional and ethical: maintain respect, patient confidentiality and cultural awareness.

comprehensive approach to the combination of risk factors for various diseases, which are much more important than individual risk factors. For example, advising a patient about his or her risk of premature cardiovascular disease will involve knowing about the patient's family history, smoking history, previous and current blood pressure, current and historical cholesterol levels, dietary history, assessment for diabetes and level of exercise undertaken.

- Ask whether the patient has undergone a screening test for colon cancer. A strong family history of carcinoma of the colon is an indication for screening colonoscopy at an age earlier than 50 years.
- Women should be asked about their family history of certain malignancies such as carcinoma of the breast or ovary, and about previous screening tests for these conditions.
- The patient's vaccination record should be reviewed regularly and brought up to date when indicated.

Personal history taking

Although personal history taking can be difficult, it can also be the most satisfying of all, since interviewing can be directly

Box 2.2
The patient's personal history

Useful questions to ask
- Where do you live (e.g. house, flat or hostel)?
- Tell me about your current work and where you have worked in the past.
- Do you get on well with people at home?
- Do you get on well with people at work?
- Do you have any financial problems?
- Are you married or have you been married?
- Could you tell me about your close relationships?
- Would you describe your marriage (or living arrangements) as happy?
- Have you been hit, kicked or physically hurt by someone (physical abuse)?
- Have you been forced to have sex (sexual abuse)?
- Would you say you have a large number of friends?
- Are you religious?
- Do you feel that you are too fat or too thin?
- Has anyone in your family had problems with psychiatric illness?
- Have you ever had a nervous breakdown?
- Have you ever had a psychiatric problem?

therapeutic for the patient. Most illnesses can induce feelings of anxiety or depression, while patients with primary psychiatric illnesses often present with physical rather than psychological symptoms. The **brain–body interaction is bidirectional** and you need to understand this as you obtain the patient's story. The patient may be reluctant or initially unable to discuss sensitive problems with a stranger, so establishing a good relationship and gaining the patient's confidence is critical (see Box 2.2).

T&O'C examination hint box

Learn to be empathic. Put yourself in the patient's place and show your empathy; for example, 'That must have been very difficult. Can you tell me how it affected you?'

A sympathetic, unhurried approach using open-ended questions will provide much information that can be systematically recorded after the interview. It is important that you maintain your matter-of-fact demeanour, particularly when asking about

Box 2.3
Symptoms of depression

Useful questions to ask
- Have you been feeling sad, down or blue?
- Have you felt depressed or lost interest in things daily for 2 or more weeks in the past?
- Have you ever felt like taking your own life?
- Do you find you wake very early in the morning?
- Has your appetite been poor recently?
- Have you lost weight recently?
- How do you feel about the future?
- Have you had trouble concentrating on things?
- Have you had guilty thoughts?
- Have you lost interest in things you usually enjoy?

Box 2.4
Symptoms of anxiety

Useful questions to ask
- Do you worry excessively about things?
- Do you have trouble relaxing?
- Do you have problems getting to sleep at night?
- Do you feel uncomfortable in crowded places?
- Do you worry excessively about minor things?
- Do you feel suddenly frightened, anxious or panicky for no reason in situations in which most people would not be afraid?
- Do you find you have to do things repetitively, such as washing your hands multiple times?
- Do you have any rituals (such as checking things) that you feel you have to do, even though you know it may be silly?
- Do you have recurrent thoughts that you have trouble controlling?

delicate subjects such as sexual problems, grief reactions or abuse.

The formal psychiatric interview differs from general medical history taking. It often takes considerable time for patients to develop rapport with, and confidence in, the clinician. There are certain standard questions that may provide valuable insight into the patient's state of mind (see Boxes 2.3 and 2.4). It may be important to obtain much more detailed information about these problems, depending on the clinical circumstances.

Depression is common in people with chronic illnesses. It is often overlooked, but it is treatable. Two simple screening questions to assess for depression are:

1. In the past month, have you felt down or hopeless?
2. Have you felt little interest or pleasure in doing things?

If the answer to one or both questions is yes, you should ask more detailed questions about depression and anxiety, including assessing for any suicidal thoughts (see Box 2.3). For example, ask:

- Have you ever thought that life was not worth living?
- Have you ever felt so bad that you have considered ending it all?

Asking about suicidal thoughts does *not* increase the risk of suicide or place the idea in the patient's mind.

Sympathetic confrontation can be helpful in difficult situations. For example, if the patient appears sad, angry or frightened, referring to this in a tactful way may lead the patient to volunteer appropriate information. If an emotional response is obtained, use emotion-handling skills (**NURS**) to deal with this during the interview (see Box 2.5).

Box 2.5
Emotion-handling skills—NURS

Name the emotion
Show **U**nderstanding
Deal with the issue with great **R**espect
Show **S**upport
For example, 'It makes sense that you were angry after your husband left you. This must have been very difficult to deal with. Can I be of any help to you now?'

Cultural history taking

Attitudes to illness and disease vary in different cultures. Problems considered shameful by the patient may be very difficult for him or her to discuss. In some cultures women may object to being, or it may not be acceptable for women to be, questioned or examined by male doctors or students. Male students may need to be accompanied by a female chaperone when interviewing female patients and should have a female chaperone when undertaking a female patient's physical examination. In some cultures, shaking hands with the opposite sex is unacceptable.

It is most important that cultural sensitivities on either side do not prevent a thorough medical assessment. If in doubt, ask the patient.

Aboriginal, Torres Strait Islander and Māori patients may have a large extended family. These relatives may be able to provide invaluable support to the patient, but the medical or social problems may interfere with the patient's ability to manage his or her own health. Commitments to family members may make it difficult for a patient to attend medical appointments or travel for specialist treatment. Detailed questioning about family contacts and responsibilities may help with planning of the patient's treatment.

MANAGING RELATIVES AND LANGUAGE PROBLEMS

- It is alarmingly common for relatives who accompany patients to interrupt and contradict the patient's (and each other's) version of events.[2]
- The interposition of a relative between the clinician and the patient always makes the history taking less direct and the patient's symptoms more subject to 'filtering' or interpretation before the information reaches the clinician. Try to sit on one side of the patient, with the relative on the other side.
- Try tactfully to direct the relative to allow the patient to answer in his or her own words, but remember that a patient with dementia may need help in providing an accurate history.
- For patients who speak little English, use of an official medical interpreter is appropriate. However, the need for an interpreter makes history taking more time-consuming and difficult.
- It is better to avoid using a patient's relative as an interpreter if possible, to reduce bias. Professional medical

2 Although a patient's deafness is sometimes given as a reason for these interruptions you may be able to overcome this problem by loud and clear speech (shouting).

translators are trained not to reinterpret the patient's history and have a good knowledge of medical terms.
- Learn to make eye contact with the patient rather than the interpreter during the interview, otherwise the patient may feel left out of the discussion.
- Questions should be directed as if going straight to the patient: 'Have you had any problems with shortness of breath?' rather than 'Has he had any breathlessness?'

T&O'C examination hint box

Assessing the patient's feelings and function using the mnemonic FIFE

Illness affects both patients and their families. Helping patients to function is part of patient management, so determining the effects of a patient's illness is key. At the end of the history it is helpful to ascertain the following:
- **F**eelings about the patient's problem
- **I**deas on what the patient believes has been occurring
- **F**unctioning—the effects of the illness on the patient
- **E**xpectations, including the patient's expectations of what the doctor will do.

Functional history taking: activities and instrumental activities of daily living

Elderly patients and patients with chronic disabling illnesses need to have their ability to manage normal living assessed. As part of the review of such a patient's symptoms, ask basic screening questions about:
- **activities of daily living** (**ADLs**), such as the patient's ability to bathe, walk, use the toilet, and eat and dress
- **instrumental activities of daily living** (**IADLs**), such as shopping, cooking and cleaning, using transport, and managing money and medications.

This assessment extends beyond medical diagnosis so that the clinician can accurately judge the patient's social and domestic circumstances. Related questions about the patient's domestic arrangements will be important if the ADLs are limited. This includes:
- number of steps in the house
- provision of railings in the bathroom

- accessibility of cupboards
- access to transport for shopping and medical treatment
- availability of help for housework and cooking
- who else lives with the patient and how those people seem to be coping with the patient's illness.

The amount of detail required depends on the severity and chronicity of the patient's illness.

Communication

Excellent communication skills are central to best clinical practice and can be learned. Communication scenarios you should master include:

- how to deliver bad news
- talking to partners or carers
- how to address a patient or relative unhappy with the medical care provided
- interacting with a patient who is blind or deaf
- interviewing a patient with a first language other than English
- how to discuss a do-not-resuscitate request.

These and other communication topics are common OSCE (objective structured clinical examination) stations.

T&O'C examination hint box

A communication framework
- Ascertain the patient's **I**deas, **C**oncerns and **E**xpectations (ICE).
- Promote empathy: see the problem from the patient's point of view and make this clear to the patient.
- Acknowledge emotion: **N**ame it, show **U**nderstanding, deal with the problems with great **R**espect and show **S**upport (NURS).

Practise your communication skills with colleagues and video your sessions to learn the pitfalls.

BREAKING BAD NEWS

'Bad news' is any information that will adversely affect a patient's view of his or her future. Patients want the truth, and ethically and legally doctors are obliged to provide this information. Breaking such news must be done with empathy and care despite the strain this causes everyone. A good mnemonic for the key steps in this process is **ABCDEF** (or alternatively, **SPIKES**):

Advance preparation (**S**etting up the interview)
- Review and know the pertinent information, find a private location and rehearse what you will say.

Build a therapeutic environment and relationship (**P**erceptions of the patient)
- Introduce yourself.
- Prepare the patient; for example, say 'I'm very sorry, but I have some bad news.'
- Ask before you tell: find out what the patient and family already know (assess their *i*deas, *c*oncerns and *e*xpectations—ICE).

Communicate (**I**nvitation to proceed)
- Agree on how much to discuss in the interview; for example, 'We have your results. Would you like us to provide all the information now?'

Deal with the patient and family (**K**nowledge provided)
- Be clear; for example, use the words 'cancer' or 'death'. Do not use jargon, code or very technical words. Avoid unnecessary bluntness.
- Go at the patient's pace. Provide information in small increments.
- Allow for silence and tears.
- Ask for the patient's understanding of what you have said.

Encourage and validate emotions (**E**motions addressed)
- Listen and observe the emotional reaction—identify the emotion (NURS).
- Give patients time to express their feelings or, if there is silence, ask what their feelings are, then reflect back (so they know you understand) by making a connecting statement such as, 'I know this is upsetting and is not what you had hoped. I wish the news were better.'
- Show support. It is often appropriate to repeat 'I am sorry'.
- Offer realistic hope.
- Provide information or say, where appropriate, 'I don't know'.

Future considered (**S**trategy for the future)
– Provide a clear plan for the next steps.[3]

The 'difficult' patient

Most clinical encounters are a cooperative effort on the part of the patient and the clinician. The patient wants help to find out what is wrong and to get better. However, interviews do not always run smoothly. **Resentment** may occur on both sides if the patient seems not to be taking the doctor's advice seriously or will not cooperate with attempts at history taking or examination. Unless there is a serious psychiatric or neurological problem that impairs the patient's judgement, this remains the patient's prerogative.

Always remember:

● As a clinician you have a duty to **give advice and explanation**, not to dictate. Indeed, it is arrogant to assume that your advice is always right. The best doctors are humble and recognise their limitations.

● Patients who seem sceptical about what they are being advised must always be given the chance to think things over and to seek other opinions. However, this approach must not be used as an excuse for not providing a proper, sympathetic and thorough explanation of the problem and the consequences of ignoring medical advice—to the extent that the patient will allow.

T&O'C examination hint box

• Patients who are **aggressive** and uncooperative may have a medical reason for their behaviour. The possibilities to be considered include alcohol or drug withdrawal, an intracranial lesion such as a tumour or subdural haematoma, or a psychiatric disease such as paranoid schizophrenia. In other cases, resentment at the occurrence of illness may be the problem.

• Urinary tract infections are a common cause of recent-onset confusion and delirium in elderly people.

---

3 Our job is 'to cure sometimes, to relieve often, to comfort always' (attributed to the American physician Edward Trudeau).

Some patients may seem difficult because they are **too cooperative**:

- The patient concerned about his blood pressure may have brought printouts of his own blood pressure measurements at half-hour intervals for several weeks. It is important to show restrained interest in these recordings without encouraging excessive enthusiasm.[4]
- Other patients may bring information about their symptoms or a diagnosis obtained from the internet. It is important to remember, and perhaps to point out, that information obtained in this way may not have been subjected to any form of peer review.

People with chronic illnesses, on the other hand, may know more about their condition than their clinician.

Sometimes the interests of the patient and the doctor are not the same. This is especially so in cases where there is the possibility of compensation for an illness or injury.

- A very small number of patients may, consciously or unconsciously, attempt to **manipulate the encounter**. This is a very difficult problem and can be approached only with rigorous application of clinical methods.
- Occasionally, attempted manipulation takes the form of flattery or inappropriate personal interest directed at the clinician. This should be dealt with by maintaining careful professional detachment. The clinician and the patient must be conscious that their meeting is strictly professional and not social.

History-taking OSCE: hints panel

The OSCE is an evaluation tool used to assess some or all of the following: history-taking skills, clinical examination skills, communication skills with patients and families, data interpretation, ability to document information, ability to infer the differential diagnosis, and technical skills. The OSCE consists of numerous stations, and students move from station to station on the same timetable, spending 10–15 minutes at each one. Each station is scored separately and scores are combined to determine the pass level.

---

4 Remember how benign this interest is compared with the enthusiasm some patients show for their gastrointestinal tract and its products.

A number of history-taking skills can be tested. A real patient or an actor may be available to answer questions and enable the examiner to test your interviewing technique and knowledge. An approach to some of these questions is summarised here as an example.

Begin all interviews by introducing yourself. In most cases the first question should probably be 'May I ask you some questions?' or 'May I have a look at you?'

1. Question this patient about her risk factors for cardiovascular disease.
   (a) Ask her the following:
      (i) How old are you?
      (ii) Do you have a previous history of cardiovascular disease or high blood pressure?
      (iii) What is your cholesterol level? (Has it been treated or untreated?)
      (iv) Do you have diabetes? (If so, for how long?)
      (v) Do you smoke? (If so, for how long? How many?)
      (vi) Do you have a family history of cardiovascular disease? (If so, who was affected and at what age?)
   (b) Synthesise and present your findings.
2. This man is short of breath. Take a history from him about this.
   (a) Ask him the following:
      (i) When are you short of breath (on exertion; lying flat—orthopnoea or paroxysmal nocturnal dyspnoea)?
      (ii) How bad is it? (Grades I–IV) Does it stop you walking up stairs or hills?
      (iii) How long does it last? Is it getting worse? Do you have any other symptoms (e.g. wheeze, chest tightness, leg swelling)?
      (iv) Do you have cough? Any sputum? (Colour?) Fever? Pleuritic chest pain?
      (v) Have you had previous heart or lung disease?
      (vi) Do you smoke? (If so, for how long? How many?)
   (b) Synthesise and present your findings.

3. This man has chronic rheumatoid arthritis. Assess his social situation.
   (a) Ask him the following:
      (i) How long have you had arthritis?
      (ii) Which joints are affected? For how long are your joints stiff in the morning?
      (iii) Can you bathe yourself, go to the toilet, dress yourself, cut food, eat? (ADLs)
      (iv) How do you manage shopping, cooking, cleaning, transport and driving, managing medications and finances? (IADLs)
      (v) Do you work?
      (vi) Who lives at home with you?
      (vii) What support do you get?
      (viii) What is the layout of your house (are there rails, steps etc)?
   (b) Synthesise and present your findings.

4. This woman has been having problems with depression. Take a history from her.
   (a) Ask her the following:
      (i) Have you been feeling sad? For how long?
      (ii) Have you felt depressed or lost interest in things daily for 2 or more weeks in the past?
      (iii) Is there any particular precipitating problem?
      (iv) Do you wake early in the mornings?
      (v) Do you suffer from loss of appetite or weight?
      (vi) What are your thoughts about the future?
      (vii) Are you able to concentrate?
      (viii) Do you have guilty thoughts?
      (ix) Have you experienced loss of interest in things you usually enjoy?
      (x) Have you ever thought of killing yourself? Have you thought what you might do?
      (xi) What treatment have you had?
      (xii) Do you have a history of major medical problems like cancer?
   (b) Synthesise and present your findings.

T&O'C examination essentials

Taking a better history

1. Ask open questions to start with (and resist the urge to interrupt), but finish with specific questions to narrow the differential diagnosis.
2. Do not hurry (or at least do not appear to be in a hurry, even if you have only limited time). It helps to have a well-practised and logical approach.
3. Ask the patient 'What else?' after he or she has finished speaking, to ensure that all problems have been identified. Repeat the 'What else?' question as often as required.
4. Keep comfortable eye contact and an open posture.
5. Use the head nod appropriately, and use silences to encourage the patient to express himself or herself.
6. When there are breaks in the narrative, provide a summary for the patient, by briefly restating the facts or feelings identified, to maximise accuracy and demonstrate active listening.
7. Clarify the list of chief or presenting complaints with the patient, rather than assuming that you know them.
8. If you are confused about the chronology of events or other issues, admit it and ask the patient to clarify. For patients with a complicated medical history it can sometimes be helpful to quickly sketch a timeline of major health (ill-health) events that have occurred during the patient's life.
9. Make sure the patient's story is consistent and, if not, ask more questions to verify the facts.
10. If emotions are uncovered, *name* the patient's emotion and indicate that you *understand* (e.g. 'you seem sad'), show *respect* and express your *support* (e.g. 'it's understandable that you would feel upset').
11. Ask about any other concerns the patient may have and address specific fears.
12. Show empathy and express your support and willingness to cooperate with the patient to help solve the problems together.

Beginning the examination

Don't touch the patient—state first what you see, cultivate your powers of observation.

Sir William Osler (1849–1919)

It is thrilling to search for objective evidence of disease (physical signs). To do this well you need to:

- develop your own systematic technique and practise this until it becomes second nature and can be performed smoothly during OSCEs and other examinations
- decide the likely diagnostic possibilities so that you can search for other clues to support or refute your differential diagnosis
- remember that common things are common so, considering the patient's age and sex, think about the most frequent possibilities first when formulating your differential diagnosis list. Hence the Zebra Rule in medicine—'when you hear hoof beats, think of horses [*common things are common*] not zebras [*rarities*]'.

Equipment

Most students equip themselves with a number of frequently used items.

- The most glamorous and arguably the most useful bedside tool (except for the only really vital tool, a pen) is the stethoscope (invented in 1816).[1] Many types are available and most work well. It is said that it is what is between the ear-pieces of the stethoscope that really matters. The stethoscope needs to be robust and easily squashed into different-sized pockets. It must also be comfortable when worn in the current fashionable position (i.e. slung around the neck). Some newer models do not have a separate bell and diaphragm. Electronic stethoscopes, which amplify sounds, are particularly helpful for students with hearing difficulties. They sound different from acoustic stethoscopes and should not be used for the first time in an exam (in fact, they are not allowed in some clinical exams).

- It is also worth acquiring a **small pocket ophthalmoscope**, a **torch** and a **short patellar hammer**. More senior students can usually give advice about the most reliable and inexpensive models available.

Most other equipment can be obtained on the wards.

Hand-washing

Patients must come first and reducing the spread of infection is your responsibility as a healthcare professional. You must wash your hands *before* touching a patient (to protect them) and *after* completing your examination (to protect you) **every time**

---

1 It is likely to disappear this century and be replaced by hand-held ultrasonography.

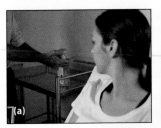
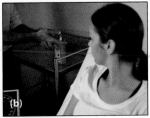
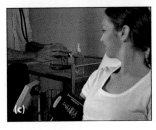

Figure 3.1 Examiner washing hands **(a and b)** and stethoscope **(c)**.

without fail. Follow the World Health Organization (WHO) guidelines:

- If there is any dirt or material on your hands, use soap and water, covering all hand surfaces for at least 40 seconds.
- If there is no soiling on your hands, use a palmful of alcohol-based formulation (alcohol rub) applied for at least 20 seconds (see Fig 3.1).
- The correct sequence is to rub:
  - hands palm to palm
  - right palm over the left dorsum with interlaced fingers, then vice versa
  - palm to palm with interlaced fingers
  - back of the fingers to opposing palms with interlocked fingers
  - each thumb rotationally
  - the palms rotationally.
- Finally, if using soap and water, rinse your hands, dry with a towel and use the towel (or your elbow) to turn off the tap. If using alcohol rub, let dry and proceed.

- Do not use alcohol rub if your hands are soiled or if there is an outbreak of *Clostridium difficile* infection; use soap and water instead.[2]

Do not forget to clean your stethoscope bell and diaphragm with an alcohol wipe after every examination.

> **T&O'C examination essentials**
>
> Correct hand-washing is not just necessary in examinations but also forms part of the student's assessment.

First impressions

Is the patient relatively well or very ill? Specific abnormalities can sometimes be recognised. Look particularly for:

- **laboured breathing**—an obvious increase in the respiratory rate and use of the accessory muscles of respiration suggest serious respiratory, cardiac or metabolic problems; this is often made more obvious when the patient mildly exerts himself or herself, such as by moving around in bed or getting undressed
- **jaundice** (yellow discolouration of the skin and sclerae)
- **cyanosis** (blue discolouration of the skin)
- **pallor** (suggesting anaemia)
- **diagnostic facies** (see Table 3.1).

TABLE 3.1   Some important diagnostic facies
ACROMEGALIC

- Prominent chin
- Supra-orbital ridges

(Smith CB, Waite PD. Surgical management of obstructive sleep apnea in acromegaly with mandibular prognathism and macroglossia: a treatment dilemma. *Journal of Oral and Maxillofacial Surgery* 2012; 70(1):207–210. © 2012. Figure 2.)

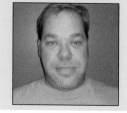

---

2 Optional if you have a death wish (if you do, please seek immediate help).

TABLE 3.1 Some important diagnostic facies *continued*

CUSHINGOID

- Plethoric and fat

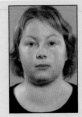

(Douglas G et al. *Macleod's Clinical Examination 13e*. Elsevier; 2013, Figure 5.16A.)

DOWN SYNDROME

- Epicanthic folds
- Large tongue

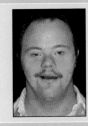

(Regezi JA et al. *Oral Pathology: Clinical Pathologic Correlations 6e*. Elsevier; 2012, Figure 15.21A.)

HIPPOCRATIC (ADVANCED PERITONITIS)

- Eyes sunken
- Temples collapsed
- Nose pinched with crusts on lips
- Forehead clammy

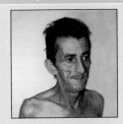

(Lemmi & Lemmi. *Physical Assessment Findings Multi-User CD-ROM*. Saunders; 2000.)

MARFANOID

- Thin, high arched palate

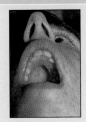

(Forbes CD, Jackson WF. *Color Atlas and Text of Clinical Medicine*. Elsevier; 2003.)

continued

TABLE 3.1 Some important diagnostic facies *continued*

MITRAL STENOSIS

- Malar flush (bluish discolouration over the cheeks)

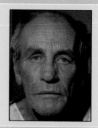

(Rehman, Habib ur, MBBS. Carcinoid syndrome. *Canadian Medical Association Journal* 2009; 180(13):1329–1329. © 2009 Canadian Medical Association.)

MYOPATHIC (DYSTROPHIA MYOTONICA)

- Frontal balding
- Triangular, wasted masseters
- Thick spectacles or intraocular lens implantation

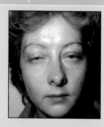

(Kanski JJ, Bowling B. *Clinical Ophthalmology: A Systematic Approach 7e.* Elsevier; 2011, Figure 19.93.)

MYXOEDEMATOUS (HYPOTHYROID)

- Puffy
- Lacking in expression
- Skin thickening
- Thinning hair
- Loss of outer one-third of eyebrows

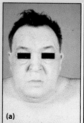
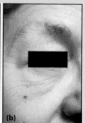

(a) (b)

(Larsen PR, Kronenberg HM, Melmed S, Polonsky KS. *Williams Textbook of Endocrinology 10e.* Philadelphia: WB Saunders; 2003, Figure 13-1AB.)

TABLE 3.1 Some important diagnostic facies *continued*

PAGETIC

- Large cranium

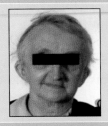

(Seton M. *Rheumatology 6e*. Elsevier;
2015, Figure 206.7.)

PARKINSONIAN

- Expressionless
- Infrequent blinking

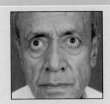

(Kanski JJ, Bowling B. *Clinical
Ophthalmology: A Systematic
Approach 7e*. Elsevier; 2011,
Figure 1.76D.)

THYROTOXIC

- Thyroid stare
- Lid retraction
- Exophthalmos

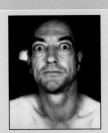

(Glynn M, Drake W. *Hutchison's
Clinical Methods: An Integrated
Approach to Clinical Practice 23e*.
Elsevier; 2012, Figure 16.13.)

VIRILE FACIES

- Acne
- Facial hair in women

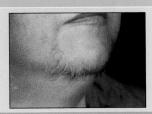

(Lebwohl MG, Heymann WR,
Berth-Jones J, Coulson I [eds].
Treatment of Skin Disease.
St Louis: Mosby; 2002.)

Check whether the patent is attached to any medical equipment such as:

- monitoring equipment (ECG, oximetry)
- supplementary oxygen (note flow rate)
- intravenous infusions (note fluid).

Vital signs

Vital signs are indicators of the function of essential parts of the body. They should be assessed in all patients at the time of the initial examination and then as often as necessary.

1. Start by examining the **radial pulse** (see Fig 3.2). It is usually palpable just medial to the distal radius with the pulps of the forefinger and middle finger of the examining hand. Count the rate over 30 seconds (and record as beats per minute; see Ch 4).

2. Measure the **blood pressure** (see Fig 3.3a).

   The normal width of the blood pressure cuff is 12.5 cm. This is suitable for a normal-sized adult upper arm. However, in obese patients with large arms, this cuff will overestimate the blood pressure and therefore a large cuff must be used. A range of smaller sizes is available for children.

   The cuff is wrapped around the patient's upper arm (which should be supported at the level of the heart) and

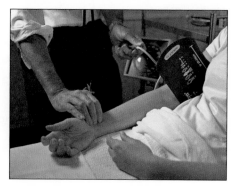

Figure 3.2 Taking the blood pressure (palpation method).

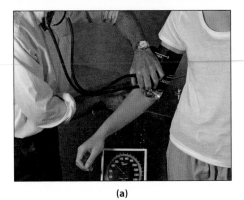

(a)

Phase	Korotkoff sounds	
		—— 120 mmHg systolic
I	A thud	
		—— 110 mmHg
II	A blowing noise	
		—— 100 mmHg
III	A softer thud	
		—— 90 mmHg diastolic (1st)
IV	A disappearing blowing noise	
		—— 80 mmHg diastolic (2nd)
V	Nothing	

(b)

Figure 3.3 **(a)** Taking the blood pressure using a cuff. **(b)** Korotkoff sounds.

the bladder centred over the brachial artery. This is found in the antecubital fossa immediately medial to the biceps tendon.

For an approximate estimation of the systolic blood pressure, the cuff is fully inflated and then deflated slowly (2 mmHg per second) until the radial pulse returns (**palpation method**). Then, for a more accurate estimation of the blood pressure, this manoeuvre is repeated with the stethoscope placed over the brachial artery (**auscultation method**). You must master both methods.

Five sounds will be heard as the cuff is slowly released (see Fig 3.3b). These are called the **Korotkoff sounds**:

- the pressure at which a sound is first heard over the artery is the systolic blood pressure (Korotkoff I [KI])
- as deflation of the cuff continues the sound increases in intensity (KII)
- then decreases (KIII)
- becomes muffled (KIV)
- and then disappears (KV). Disappearance is normally taken to indicate the level of the diastolic pressure. A normal **auscultatory gap** may sometimes occur (the sounds disappear just below systolic pressure but reappear above diastolic).

The systolic blood pressure may normally vary between the arms by up to 10 mmHg; in the legs, where it can be taken with a special large cuff placed over the thigh (the popliteal artery is used instead of the brachial), the blood pressure is normally higher than in the arms (this measurement is not routine). However, if coarctation of the aorta or subclavian artery stenosis is suspected, these readings may be performed.

A classification of blood pressure readings

- **Optimal** blood pressure: <120 mmHg systolic; <80 mmHg diastolic.
- **High normal** blood pressure: 130–139 mmHg systolic; and/or 85–89 mmHg diastolic.
- **Mild hypertension (grade 1):** 140–159 mmHg systolic; and/or 90–99 mmHg diastolic.
- **Moderate hypertension (grade 2):** 160–179 mmHg systolic; and/or 100–109 mmHg diastolic.
- **Severe hypertension (grade 3):** ≥180 mmHg systolic; and /or ≥110 mmHg diastolic.

Blood pressure measured at home by the patient or with a 24-hour monitor will confirm surgery readings that may be artificially high (**white-coat hypertension**, so-called because doctors all used to wear white coats).

During inspiration, the systolic and diastolic blood pressures normally decrease. When this normal reduction in blood pressure with inspiration is exaggerated (more than 10 mmHg), it is termed **pulsus paradoxus**. Causes include constrictive pericarditis, pericardial effusion and severe asthma. To measure pulsus paradoxus:

- lower the cuff slowly and note when the KI sound is occurring intermittently (expiration)
- lower the cuff further until KI is audible with every beat: the difference equals the pulsus paradoxus.

3. Take the **temperature**.
   - Electronic thermometers have replaced mercury ones in hospitals. The temperature is taken in the ear and the device beeps in a helpful way when ready.
   - The normal temperature is 37°C if taken in the mouth or ear; it is about 1°C less if taken in the axilla and about 1°C more if taken in the rectum.

4. Count the **respiratory rate**.
   - The normal rate is between 16 and 25 breaths per minute.
   - An increased rate may be due to lung disease of almost any type, cardiac failure or metabolic disturbances such as acidosis, or psychological conditions such as anxiety.

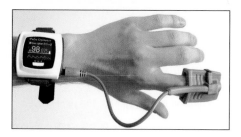

Figure 3.4   Pulse oximeter.

5. Use pulse oximetry to measure the patient's arterial blood oxygen saturation (SpO_2).
    - The device is placed on the ear lobe or finger (see Fig 3.4).
    - A falsely low reading may occur as a result of coloured nail polish or reduced tissue perfusion due to cold.
    - A reading of >95% is generally considered normal.
    - A reading of <90% is very abnormal and may indicate respiratory failure.

General appearance

Before specifically examining the regions or medical systems of the body, a general inspection must be made. Make a conscious effort and take the time to consider the patient's appearance, including:

- **face** (see Table 3.1)
- **hands** (see Table 3.2)
- **body**.

Certain facies and body habituses are diagnostic or nearly so. Important relevant signs may be missed unless this is done (seeing the wood rather than the trees). For example, a patient with weight loss may not be identified as having thyrotoxicosis (see Ch 9) unless the eye signs (e.g. thyroid stare) are noticed.

Weight and body habitus

1. Look specifically for:
    - obesity
    - wasting (loss of muscle mass)
    - an unusual facial appearance (see Table 3.1)
    - abnormal body shape (e.g. the tall, thin appearance with long fingers that occurs in Marfan's syndrome).

TABLE 3.2 Nail signs in systemic disease

Nail sign	Some causes	Example
Clubbing	Lung cancer, cyanotic congenital heart disease, endocarditis, inflammatory bowel disease, cirrhosis (Zipes DP et al. *Braunwald's Heart Disease: A Textbook of Cardiovascular Medicine 7e.* Philadelphia: Saunders; 2005.)	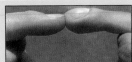
Koilonychia (spoon-shaped nails)	Iron deficiency anaemia (James DW. *Andrews' Diseases of the Skin.* Elsevier 2011, Figure 33.41.)	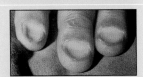
Onycholysis (separation of nail from nail bed)	Psoriasis, infection, hyperthyroidism, trauma (Bernard A, Cohen MD. *Pediatric Dermatology 4e.* © 2013, Elsevier Limited, Figure 8.67.)	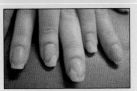
Pitting	Psoriasis, Reiter's syndrome (Bolognia J et al. *Dermatology 3e.* Elsevier; 2012, Figure 71.4.)	
Beau's lines	Any severe systemic illness that disrupts nail growth, Raynaud's disease, pemphigus, trauma (Habif TP. *Clinical Dermatology: A Color Guide to Diagnosis and Therapy,* Elsevier; 2010, Figure 14-13.)	
Yellow nails	Lymphoedema, pleural effusion, immunodeficiency, bronchiectasis, sinusitis, rheumatoid arthritis, nephrotic syndrome, thyroiditis, tuberculosis, Raynaud's disease (*American Journal of Medicine* 2010; 123(2):125–126, Elsevier, Figure 2.)	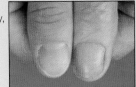

continued

TABLE 3.2   Nail signs in systemic disease   *continued*

Nail sign	Some causes	Example
Terry's (white) nails	Cirrhosis, malnutrition	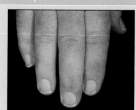
		(Callen JP, Jorizzo JL, Bolognia JL, Piette WW, Zone JJ. *Dermatological Signs of Internal Disease.* Elsevier, 2009, Figure 26-5.)
Azure lunula (blue nails)	Hepatolenticular degeneration (Wilson's disease), silver poisoning	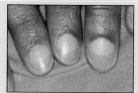
		(Naylor EMT, Ruben ES, Robinson-Bostom L, Telang GH, Jellinek NJ. *Journal of the American Academy of Dermatology* 2008; 58(6):1021–1024. Copyright © 2008 American Academy of Dermatology, Inc., Figure 1.)
Half-and-half nails	Chronic kidney disease	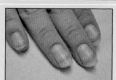
		(Schwarzenberger K, Werchniak AE, Ko CJ. *General Dermatology.* © 2009, Elsevier Limited, Figure 2-5.)
Muehrcke's lines	Hypoalbuminaemia (any cause)	
		(Short N, Shah C. *American Journal of Medicine* 2010; 123(11):991–992. Copyright © 2010 Elsevier Inc.)
Mees' lines	Arsenic poisoning, Hodgkin's lymphoma, chemotherapy	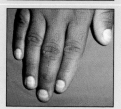
		(Chauhan S, D'Cruz S, Singh R, Sachdev A. *The Lancet* 2008; 372(9647):1410–1410. Copyright © 2008 Elsevier.)

TABLE 3.2 Nail signs in systemic disease *continued*

Nail sign	Some causes	Example
Dark longitudinal streaks	Melanoma, benign naevus, chemical staining	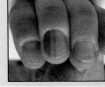
	(Piraccini BM, Dika E, Fanti PA. Tips for diagnosis and treatment of nail pigmentation with practical algorithm. *Dermatologic Clinics.* Copyright © 2015 Elsevier Inc., Figure 20.)	
Longitudinal striations	Alopecia areata, vitiligo, atopic dermatitis, psoriasis	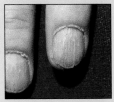
	(Paller AS, Mancini AJ. *Hurwitz Clinical Pediatric Dermatology.* Elsevier, Figure 7.54.)	
Splinter haemorrhages	Subacute bacterial endocarditis, SLE, rheumatoid arthritis, antiphospholipid syndrome, trauma	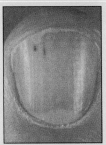
	(Forbes & Jackson. *Color Atlas and Text of Clinical Medicine 3e.* Elsevier; 2002.)	
Telangiectasia	Rheumatoid arthritis, SLE, dermatomyositis, scleroderma	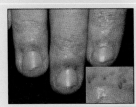
	(Bolognia JL et al. *Dermatology.* Elsevier, Figure 42.1. Courtesy Julie V Schaffer, MD.)	

SLE, systemic lupus erythematosus.

2. **Weigh** the patient.
   - For children, the height should also be measured and a weight–height chart consulted to determine the child's growth percentile.
   - For adults whose weight appears abnormal, the **body mass index (BMI)** should be calculated. The formula is weight/height squared (kg/m^2). A BMI between 18.5 and 25 is normal, while ≥30 indicates obesity and <18.5 indicates underweight.

3. Measure the **waist circumference** (a measure of abdominal obesity).
   - Find the upper hip bone and top of the iliac crest and place the measuring tape around the abdomen at the level of the iliac crest.
   - For women, >80 cm indicates an increased health risk and >88 cm a greatly increased risk.
   - For men, >94 cm indicates an increased health risk and >102 cm a greatly increased risk.

4. Inspect for **limb deformity** or missing limbs (these are not always obvious if the patient is huddled under the bedclothes). If the patient walks into the examining room, the opportunity to examine walking (gait) should not be lost; the full testing of gait is described in Chapter 7.

5. Assess the state of **hydration**.
   - Severe dehydration is associated with sunken orbits, dry mucous membranes (e.g. look at the tongue), reduced skin elasticity (turgor—an area of skin when pulled away from the body hangs in a wrinkled state for some seconds before falling back) and hypotension (low blood pressure).

6. Look for **pallor**, which may indicate anaemia, and for a blue tongue (and blue fingers), which may indicate central cyanosis, a sign of arterial oxygen desaturation (see p. 76).

The hands and nails

Examination of a system of the body often begins with inspection of the hands and nails. For example, the patient with suspected chronic liver disease may have:
- **liver nails** (white nail beds with a rim of pink at the top)
- **palmar erythema** (red palms).

Nail and finger changes may also occur in cardiac and respiratory diseases, endocrine diseases, arthritis and anaemia (see Table 3.2).

How to examine a lump

Lumps may be present anywhere on the surface of the body. They are usually readily examined and you must have an approach that helps work out the cause. Ask whether a lump is painful before you palpate it.

1. After washing your hands, look at and feel the lump to work out:
   - anatomical site on the body
   - size
   - shape and contour (e.g. well defined or irregular)
   - colour (e.g. pigmented—naevus, re-inflammation)
   - consistency (soft or hard—enlarged lymph nodes often feel 'rubbery' when they are caused by a lymphoma)
   - tenderness or not.
2. Next, work out in what tissue layer the lump is situated.
   - If it is in the **skin** (e.g. sebaceous cyst, epidermoid cyst, papilloma), it should move when the skin is moved.
   - If it is in **subcutaneous tissue** (e.g. neurofibroma, lipoma), the skin can be moved over the lump.
   - If it is in a **muscle** or **tendon** (e.g. tumour), then contraction of the muscle or tendon will limit the lump's mobility; mobility is greater in the transverse than the longitudinal axis.
   - If it is in a **nerve**, pressing on the lump may result in pins and needles (paraesthesias) being felt in the distribution of the nerve, and the lump cannot be moved in the longitudinal axis but can be moved in the transverse axis.
   - If it is in **bone**, the lump will be immobile.
   - If it is arising from an artery, it will be pulsatile.
3. Find out whether the lump is **fluctuant** (i.e. contains fluid; see Fig. 3.5).
   - Place two forefingers (the 'watching' fingers) halfway between the centre and periphery of the lump.
   - Place the forefinger from the other hand (the 'displacing' finger) diagonally opposite at an equal distance from the centre of the lump.

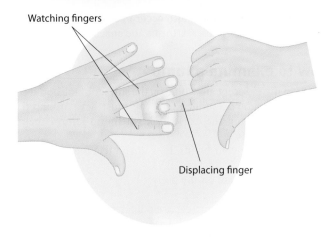

Watching fingers

Displacing finger

Figure 3.5   Testing a lump for fluctuation.

- Press with the displacing finger and keep the watching fingers still. If the lump contains fluid, the watching fingers will be displaced in **both** axes of the lump (i.e. fluctuation is present).
- Place a small torch behind the lump to determine whether it can be **transilluminated** (if there is fluid, light will shine through the lump).

4. Note any **associated signs of inflammation** (i.e. redness, swelling, heat and tenderness).
5. Look for **similar lumps elsewhere** (e.g. multiple subcutaneous swellings from neurofibromas or lipomas). If an inflammatory or neoplastic lump is suspected, remember always to examine the regional **lymphatic field** and the other lymph node groups, as explained in Chapter 6.

Always remember to describe a lump:

• Site	• Consistency	• Tenderness
• Size	• Colour	• Tethering
• Shape	• Contour	• Temperature

Preparing the patient for examination

Try to ensure that the patient is comfortable and positioned so as to assist the examination. Every effort should be made to ensure that the examination is not uncomfortable or embarrassing. The curtains should be drawn around the bed and members of the clinician's entourage should be introduced. At each stage the patient should be informed about what is going to happen.

- Wash and make an effort to warm your examining hands and stethoscope before they are applied to the patient's skin. Always wash your hands before and after touching a patient to protect the patient and yourself.
- The patient must be undressed so that the parts to be examined are accessible.
- Modesty requires that a woman's breasts be covered temporarily with a gown or sheet while other parts of the body are being examined.
- Men and women should both have the groin covered; for example, during examination of the legs. However, important physical signs will be missed in some patients if excessive attention is paid to modesty.
- The position of the patient in bed or elsewhere should depend on what is to be examined. For example, a patient's abdomen is best examined if he or she lies completely flat so that the abdominal muscles are relaxed.
- Traditionally, the doctor examines from the right side of the bed.

Beginning the examination OSCE: hints panel

This OSCE may involve important spot diagnoses or demonstration of important examination techniques. The examiner will usually give a very specific instruction about what is to be done. It is important to listen carefully to any introduction given about the patient. These introductions (often a brief history) are meant to help with the diagnosis.

- Always perform exactly the examination requested, but begin by introducing yourself and asking the patient's permission for you to perform the examination. For example, 'My name is Jane Fowler and I have been asked to examine your chest. Is that alright? Can I get you to sit up please and take off your shirt?'
- **Be seen to wash your hands.**
- Stand back and make a brief inspection of the whole patient.

- Some diagnoses are more obvious from a distance and important clues such as an intravenous cannula containing antibiotics or anticoagulant may otherwise be missed.

1. Take this patient's blood pressure.
   (a) Make sure you take the blood pressure by palpation and then auscultation using proper technique.
   (b) Check for a postural blood pressure drop (lying and sitting).
   (c) If the blood pressure is elevated, look for secondary causes of hypertension (e.g. palpate for radiofemoral delay in coarctation of the aorta, listen for a renal bruit, palpate for enlarged kidneys).
   (d) Look for complications of hypertension (e.g. fundoscopy changes of malignant hypertension) and cardiac failure.
   Note: There are different types of sphygmomanometer.
   Practise taking blood pressure readings with a number of different manual machines. Make sure you use the correct-sized cuff.
2. Examine this patient's fingernails; he is a smoker who has had recent lung problems.
   This introduction suggests that the abnormality may be clubbing, possibly due to carcinoma of the lung.
   (a) Stand back to look for dyspnoea or cyanosis.
   (b) Inspect the nails (see Table 3.2) from the side. Look for loss of the hyponychial angle.
   (c) Note cyanosis.
   (d) Look for tar staining.
   (e) Examine the respiratory system (p. 108).

Alternative clinical assessment tools

- In the **traditional long case**, the candidate takes the full history, performs a complete examination and determines the provisional diagnoses in priority order and a management plan. The candidate's case assessment may or may not be directly observed by the examiners. The candidate presents the case to the examiners, who then ask questions that test clinical and diagnostic skills.
- The **Objective Structured Long Examination Record (OSLER)** is an alternative to the traditional long case with an OSCE format that is more comprehensive.
- In the **traditional short case**, the candidate has 10–15 minutes to examine a system or part of the body as directed by the examiners, present the findings (positive signs and pertinent negatives) and discuss the provisional diagnosis. This testing may include spot diagnoses (identifying the major abnormality and likely disease or diagnosis on first looking at the patient).
- The **Mini-Clinical Evaluation eXercise (mini-CEX)** is a short observed patient interaction testing not only history and physical examination but also communication skills and behaviours.

T&O'C examination essentials

1. Many diagnostic clues will be missed unless time is taken to make a general inspection of the patient.
2. Always ask yourself when you see a patient, 'Is this person very unwell? Are urgent assessment and treatment needed?'
3. Always wash your hands and clean your equipment before touching a patient.
4. Always make sure that the patient is comfortable and protected from pain and embarrassment during your examination.
5. Simple procedures like measuring the blood pressure are often poorly performed by students who have not practised them. This can lead to intense embarrassment during OSCEs.
6. Wash your hands after you have completed your examination.

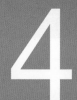

The heart and cardiovascular system

Never forget to look at the back of a patient. Always look at the feet. Looking at a woman's legs has often saved her life.

Sir William Osler (1849–1919)

This chapter presents an introduction to history taking and examination of the cardiovascular system. It is usual to begin the examination with an assessment of the peripheral signs of cardiovascular disease, as set out below. Learn to run through these questions quickly so that you can assess patients seen in clinics, on the wards or in examination long cases.

The cardiovascular system assessment sequence

1. Presenting symptoms (e.g. chest pain, dyspnoea, palpitations, peripheral oedema)
2. Detailed questions about presenting symptoms (SOCRATES)
3. Questions about previous cardiac problems and cardiac risk factors (past, social and family history)
4. A general inspection of the patient
5. Examination for peripheral signs of cardiovascular disease, including the pulses and blood pressure
6. Examination of the neck (carotid pulse and jugular venous pressure)
7. Examination of the praecordium including the apex beat, heart sounds and murmurs
8. Examination of the lung fields for signs of cardiac failure
9. Examination of the legs for oedema
10. Provisional and differential diagnosis

The cardiac history

PRESENTING SYMPTOMS (see Box 4.1)

Chest pain

Ask the patient with chest pain about:

- site (e.g. central chest)
- onset (e.g. typically with exertion or emotion, if angina)
- character (crushing tight or heavy pain is typical of angina)

Box 4.1
The cardiovascular history

Major symptoms
Chest pain, tightness, discomfort or heaviness
Dyspnoea: exertional (note degree of exercise necessary),
    orthopnoea, paroxysmal nocturnal dyspnoea
Ankle swelling
Palpitations
Syncope and dizziness
Intermittent claudication
Fatigue

Past history
Rheumatic fever, chorea, recent (past 3 months) dental work, thyroid
    disease
Prior medical examination revealing heart disease (e.g. military,
    school, insurance)
Drugs

Social history
Smoking habits and alcohol use

Family history
Myocardial infarcts, cardiomyopathy, congenital heart disease, mitral
    valve prolapse, Marfan's syndrome

Coronary artery disease risk factors
Previous coronary or vascular disease
Hyperlipidaemia
Hypertension
Smoking
Family history of coronary artery disease
Diabetes mellitus
Obesity and physical inactivity
Male sex and advanced age

- radiation (may travel to the left arm or jaw if angina)
- alleviating factors (e.g. rest with angina)
- timing (may be brief)
- exacerbating factors (e.g. exercise if angina)
- severity (grade).

These same questions are used to assess pain anywhere in the body.

Typical ischaemic chest pain is due to inadequate blood supply to the myocardium.

- It is often described as a central or retrosternal (behind the sternum) discomfort rather than a pain.
- There is frequently a tight or heavy sensation, which may radiate to the left arm or to the jaw. It tends to occur on exertion and may be predictable at certain levels of activity.
- It may be associated with dyspnoea.
- Relief is usually rapid with rest or sublingual (under the tongue) nitrate drugs.
- Prolonged ischaemic-type pain or discomfort that comes on at rest is more suggestive of myocardial infarction than angina.
- Patients who have had the pain before usually recognise it when it occurs again.
- The pain of infarction is more likely to be associated with nausea and sweating than is the pain of angina.

Consult Table 4.1 for other causes of chest pain.

T&O'C examination essentials: Chest pain

Important differential diagnoses
- Myocardial ischaemia—infarction, angina
- Pericarditis
- Pleurisy
- Aortic dissection
- Musculoskeletal pain
- Oesophageal reflux or spasm
- Pulmonary embolism
- Pneumonia

TABLE 4.1   Causes of chest pain and typical features

Pain	Typical features
Cardiac pain	Angina (exertional), myocardial ischaemia or infarction (persistent)
Vascular pain	Aortic dissection (very sudden onset, radiates to the back)
Pleuropericardial pain	Pericarditis (pleuritic pain, worse when patient lies down) Infective pleurisy (pleuritic pain, increases on inspiration) Pneumothorax (sudden onset, sharp, associated with dyspnoea) Pneumonia (often pleuritic, associated with fever and dyspnoea) Autoimmune disease (pleuritic) Mesothelioma (severe and constant) Metastatic tumour (severe and constant, localised)
Chest wall pain	Persistent cough (worse with movement, chest wall tender) Muscular strains (worse with movement, chest wall tender) Intercostal myositis (worse with movement, chest wall tender) Thoracic herpes zoster (severe, follows nerve root distribution, precedes rash) Coxsackie B virus infection (pleuritic) Thoracic nerve compression or infiltration (follows nerve root distribution) Rib fracture (history of trauma, localised tenderness) Rib tumour, primary or metastatic (constant, severe, localised) Tietze's syndrome (costal cartilage tender)
Gastrointestinal pain	Gastro-oesophageal reflux (not related to exertion, burning, rises up towards the neck, may be worse when patient lies down) Diffuse oesophageal spasm (rare, not exertional)
Airway pain	Tracheitis (pain in throat, breathing painful) Inhaled foreign body (stridor)
Other causes	Panic attacks (often preceded by anxiety, associated with breathlessness)

1. What is the pain like? (You may need to help by asking, 'Is it heavy, tight, burning or sharp?')
2. Where is it and does it go anywhere else? (Myocardial ischaemia often causes pain or discomfort that radiates to the arm or jaw, or both. Aortic dissection often causes severe pain that radiates to the back.)
3. Is it severe?
4. How long does it last? (Pain only during exertion suggests angina or aortic stenosis. Prolonged pain at rest suggests myocardial infarction, but very prolonged pain (days) suggests something else)
5. When does it occur? (During exertion suggests angina; during the night when lying flat suggests oesophageal reflux)
6. Are there associated symptoms like sweating or nausea? (Myocardial infarction)
7. Is it painful to breathe (pleurisy) and better when you sit up (pericarditis)?
8. Have you had angina or reflux before? If so, is this the same?
9. Have you injured yourself recently? (Musculoskeletal)
10. Are you very breathless? Did this begin very suddenly? (Pulmonary embolism)
11. Have you had a cough or fever? (Pneumonia)
12. Is it relieved by rest? (Angina)
13. Is it relieved by antacids? (Oesophageal reflux)

Dyspnoea

Cardiac dyspnoea can be difficult to distinguish from that due to other causes, such as lung disease (see Table 4.2).[1]

Shortness of breath may be due to multiple causes:

- **Cardiac disease** (heart failure)—in this case, it is often associated with:
  - orthopnoea (breathlessness that is worse when the patient lies flat)

---

1 Chest physicians have been known to blame the heart for dyspnoea while cardiologists may blame the lungs: specialist 'ping pong'. You need to try to decide based on all the evidence from the clinical evaluation.

TABLE 4.2   History of dyspnoea: heart versus lungs

Favours heart failure	Favours lung disease
History of heart failure or infarction	History of smoking >10 packet years
History of valvular heart disease	History of asthma
Orthopnoea	Dust exposure
Paroxysmal nocturnal dyspnoea	History of lung disease
	Wheezing
	Relief with bronchodilators
	Cough
	Fever

- – paroxysmal nocturnal dyspnoea (PND), breathlessness that wakes the patient from sleep—typically the patient gets up and walks to the window to breathe in fresh air, and it takes several minutes for relief to occur
- **Valvular heart disease** versus **angina**—in this case:
  - – patients with valvular heart disease usually describe symptoms that are predictable with exertion but do not have orthopnoea unless heart failure has supervened
  - – when it is due to angina, dyspnoea is often associated with a feeling of chest tightness.

Ankle swelling

Peripheral oedema may be a symptom (and sign) of cardiac failure, but there are other more common causes of ankle swelling (e.g. varicose veins, vasodilating drugs).

T&O'C examination essentials: Ankle oedema

Important differential diagnoses
- Venous disease of the legs
- Calcium antagonist drugs used for hypertension
- Cardiac failure
- Lymphoedema
- Nephrotic syndrome (kidney disease)

Questions box 4.2 What to ask the patient with
ankle oedema

1. How far up your leg does the oedema extend? Do you have
   trouble putting your shoes on?
2. Are your ankles normal in the morning when you
   get up? (Lymphoedema causes persistent swelling)
3. Have you had trouble with the veins in your legs?
   Have you had surgery to treat varicose veins?
4. Do you take blood pressure tablets? If so, which
   ones?
5. Have you had heart failure or been told your heart is
   enlarged?
6. Do you get out of breath easily or at night when you lie
   down (Orthopnoea—heart failure)
7. Have you had problems with your kidneys?
8. Have you had bad problems with your lungs? (Right
   heart failure secondary to chronic lung disease—cor
   pulmonale)

Palpitations

This is usually taken to mean an unexpected awareness of the
heartbeat. Try to find out precisely what it is that the patient is
aware of. Ask about:

- the perceived heart rate
- the suddenness of onset and offset
- the regularity or irregularity of the heartbeat.

It may help to ask the patient to tap out the rhythm of the heartbeat with their fingers.

T&O'C examination essentials: Palpitations

Important differential diagnoses

- Awareness of sinus rhythm or sinus tachycardia
- Ectopic beats
- Atrial fibrillation (AF)
- Atrial flutter
- Supraventricular tachycardia (SVT)
- Ventricular tachycardia (VT)

Questions box 4.3   What to ask the patient
with palpitations

1. What do you mean by palpitations?
2. Does your heartbeat seem fast?
3. How fast? Have you tried to count it?
4. Does it seem faster than it has gone before? (SVT or VT)
5. Does it seem fast and irregular (all over the place)? (AF)
6. Does it start and stop very suddenly (like a light going on or off)? (SVT)
7. Can you make it stop by holding your breath? (SVT)
8. How long does it last?
9. How often does it happen?
10. Do you feel unwell or dizzy during episodes? (VT a little more likely)
11. Have you had damage to your heart—a heart attack in the past? (VT more likely)
12. Have you had an overactive thyroid? (Sinus tachycardia or AF)
13. Does your heart seem to miss and thump hard? (Ectopic beats)
14. Is it worse when you are resting quietly or trying to go to sleep? (Ectopic beats)
15. Is it worse before exams? (Sinus tachycardia or ectopic beats in a medical student)
16. Does it come on with exercise? (Some patients with SVT or AF)
17. Does it occur after you have large amounts of alcohol? (AF)
18. Has an episode ever been recorded on an ECG?

Syncope and dizziness

Syncope is a **transient loss of consciousness** resulting from cerebral anoxia. It is necessary to establish:

- whether the patient actually loses consciousness
- under what circumstances the syncope occurs (e.g. **postural** syncope occurs on standing, **micturition** syncope occurs when the patient is passing urine, **tussive** syncope occurs with coughing and **vasovagal** syncope occurs with sudden emotional strain).

The differential diagnosis includes **epilepsy**, where there may be associated tonic and clonic jerks (rhythmical contraction and relaxation of muscle groups). Aortic stenosis (p. 80) or hypertrophic cardiomyopathy (p. 90) may be associated with syncope that occurs on exertion.

Dizziness that occurs even when the patient is lying down or that is made worse by movements of the head is more likely to be of neurological or middle ear origin. The subjective sensation that the world is turning around suggests **vertigo**, which can be due to vestibular abnormalities (e.g. labyrinthitis).

Intermittent claudication

A history of claudication (pain in the calves when walking a certain distance) suggests peripheral vascular disease causing an inadequate arterial blood supply to the affected muscles.

Fatigue

Fatigue is a common symptom of cardiac failure but there are many other causes of this symptom, including:

- lack of sleep
- anaemia
- depression
- hypothyroidism.

RISK FACTORS FOR ATHEROSCLEROTIC CARDIAC DISEASE

1. *Ischaemic heart disease.* The most important traditional risk factors for ischaemic heart disease are:
   - diabetes mellitus
   - hyperlipidaemia
   - smoking
   - a family history of coronary artery disease (first-degree relatives—siblings or parents—affected before the age of 55 in males and 65 in females)
   - hypertension
   - male sex
   - old age.[2]

   Other risk factors include obesity, lack of exercise, more than moderate alcohol consumption and chronic kidney disease. A previous myocardial infarction, angina, stroke or peripheral vascular disease suggests underlying atherosclerosis.

2. *Valvular heart disease.*
   - A history of rheumatic fever places patients at risk of rheumatic valvular heart disease (usually aortic and mitral stenosis or regurgitation).

---

2 Can't do much about this though.

- Valvular and cardiac abnormalities are a feature of certain inherited conditions.
- Marfan's syndrome can be a cause of valve disease (e.g. aortic regurgitation, mitral valve prolapse) and aortic disease (e.g. aortic dissection).
- Down syndrome is associated with atrial septal defects (a hole in the atrium) and mitral and tricuspid valve abnormalities.
3. *A family history of cardiac muscle abnormalities.* Some forms of dilated cardiomyopathy, a cause of heart failure, and cases of hypertrophic cardiomyopathy are inherited conditions. The disease severity may differ in different families.
4. *Sudden death and cardiac arrhythmias.* Inherited abnormalities of cardiac ion transport such as the long QT interval syndrome and the Brugada syndrome (right bundle branch block pattern with septal ST elevation on the electrocardiogram) are associated with an increased risk of sudden death.

TREATMENT HISTORY

This includes:
- current and past drug treatment
- cardiac surgical history (coronary bypass grafting or valve surgery)[3]
- any history of coronary artery angioplasty or balloon valvotomy.

SOCIAL HISTORY

Social history is relevant for patients with a chronic illness and must be recorded. The availability of family and financial support is important for any patient with a serious illness and may affect such things as how soon the patient can go home.

Many cardiac conditions affect a patient's ability to work:
- heavy physical work may not be possible following an infarct or valve surgery

---

3 Patients often know how many bypasses or stents they have received and find this an opportunity for boasting.

- certain occupations (e.g. commercial flying or vehicle driving) are precluded in patients with certain heart diseases if there is an increased risk of syncope or sudden death.

Examination anatomy

The mechanical function of the heart results in movement that is often palpable (see Fig 4.10 later in the chapter) and sometimes visible on the part of the chest that lies in front of it—the praecordium. The passage of blood through the heart and its valves (see Figs 4.1 and 4.2) and on into the great vessels of the body produces many interesting sounds and causes pulsation in arteries and movement in veins in remote parts of the body. Signs of cardiac disease may be found by examining the praecordium and the many accessible arteries and veins of the body (see Fig 4.3).

Examining the heart

Examination of the cardiovascular system usually begins with a general inspection followed by a search for the peripheral signs of heart and vascular disease (see Box 4.2). It is important to begin with the patient lying in bed with enough pillows or with the bed aligned to support him or her at 45° (see Fig 4.4).

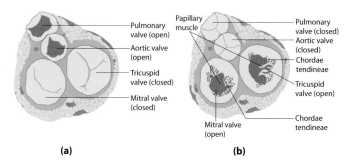

Figure 4.1 The cardiac valves in **(a)** systole and **(b)** diastole.

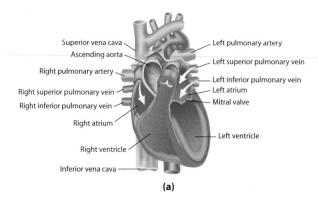

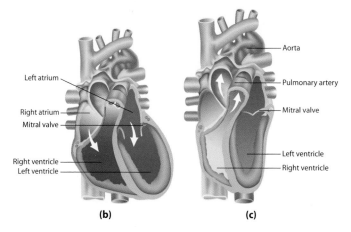

Figure 4.2   The cardiac cycle. **(a)** Early diastole—ventricles begin to relax. **(b)** Late diastole—ventricles fill. **(c)** Systole—ventricles contract.

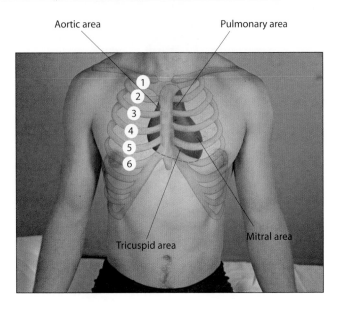

Figure 4.3 Surface anatomy of the heart. The first palpable rib is the second (2).

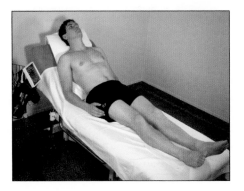

Figure 4.4 The cardiovascular examination with the patient lying at 45° and suitably undressed.

Box 4.2
The cardiovascular examination sequence

1. A general inspection of the patient
2. A search for the peripheral signs of heart and vascular disease in the arms, face and neck
   - hands and nails
   - radial pulse
   - blood pressure
   - face
   - neck
3. The praecordium
   - inspection
   - palpation
   - auscultation
   - dynamic manoeuvres
4. The back
   - percussion
   - auscultation
5. The abdomen
   - the liver
   - ascites
   - the spleen
6. The legs
   - palpation of the peripheral pulses
   - inspection for oedema and signs of arterial and venous disease

In this position the chest is easily accessible and this is the usual position in which the jugular venous pressure (JVP) is assessed (p. 77).

T&O'C examination hint box

As always, patient examinations must begin with a general inspection.

GENERAL APPEARANCE

1. If the patient walks into the clinic or you walk into the examination room, look for signs of breathlessness and any abnormality of body habitus. If the patient is in bed in hospital, also look for the use of supplemental oxygen, a cardiac ECG monitor and the presence of intravenous or arterial cannulas.

2. Note whether the patient looks well or unwell.
   - Look to see if the patient has *rapid and laboured respiration*, suggesting dyspnoea, which is both a symptom and a sign. Dyspnoea may be present as the patient undresses or even at rest.
   - Look for *cachexia*—that is, severe loss of weight and muscle wasting. This is commonly caused by malignant disease but severe cardiac failure may also produce this appearance (**cardiac cachexia**).
   - Pallor may be present as a result of anaemia. Anaemia will make the symptoms of heart failure or angina worse.
   - Cyanosis may be a sign of congenital heart disease or greatly reduced cardiac output.

THE PERIPHERAL SIGNS OF HEART DISEASE

The hands

Pick up the patient's right hand, then the left.

1. Look for **peripheral cyanosis**, which is blue discolouration of the fingers, toes and other peripheral parts of the body.
2. Look at the nails from the side for **clubbing** (see Table 3.2). This is an increase in the soft tissue of the distal part of the fingers or toes and occurs in cyanotic congenital heart disease.
3. Look for **splinter haemorrhages** in the nail beds. These are linear haemorrhages lying parallel to the long axis of the nail (see Table 3.2). They are most often due to trauma, particularly in manual workers. However, an important cause is infective endocarditis, which is a bacterial (or less commonly a fungal) infection of the heart valves or part of the endocardium.
4. **Tendon xanthomata** are yellow or orange deposits of lipid in the tendons, including those of the hand and arm. They occur in hyperlipidaemia.

T&O'C examination hint box

A patient seen for a clinical examination is unlikely to have endocarditis unless an intravenous cannula or line is in place for the administration of antibiotics.

TABLE 4.3   The character of the arterial pulse

Type of pulse	Cause(s)
Anacrotic Small volume, slow uptake, notched wave on upstroke	Aortic stenosis
Plateau Slow upstroke	Aortic stenosis
Bisferiens Anacrotic and collapsing	Aortic stenosis and regurgitation
Collapsing	Aortic regurgitation Hyperdynamic circulation Patent ductus arteriosus Peripheral arteriovenous fistula Arteriosclerotic aorta (elderly patients in particular)
Small volume	Aortic stenosis Pericardial effusion
Pulsus paradoxus	Tamponade or severe asthma

The arterial pulse (see Table 4.3)

The following observations should be made at the radial pulse:

- rate of pulse
- rhythm
- if there is a history of hypertension, the presence or absence of delay of the femoral pulse compared with the radial pulse (radiofemoral delay—a sign of coarctation of the aorta, which is a cause of upper limb hypertension; see Fig 4.5).

Rate of pulse

The pulse rate can be counted over 30 seconds and multiplied by two.[4] The normal resting heart rate in adults is between 60 and 100 beats per minute.

- **Bradycardia** is defined as a heart rate less than 60 beats per minute.
- **Tachycardia** is defined as a heart rate over 100 beats per minute.

---

4   A phone app is now available to help with this calculation.

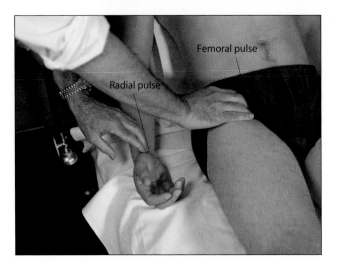

Figure 4.5 Feeling for radiofemoral delay.

Rhythm

The rhythm of the pulse can be **regular** or **irregular**. An irregular rhythm can be:

- completely *irregular with no pattern*; this is usually due to atrial fibrillation, which occurs when coordinated contraction of the atria is lost and the ventricles beat irregularly and usually fast. The pulse rate is then usually rapid (greater than 120 beats per minute) unless the patient is being treated with drugs to slow it down. An irregularly irregular pulse can occasionally be caused by frequent, irregularly occurring supraventricular or ventricular ectopic beats (extrasystoles).
- *regularly irregular*; for example, in sinus arrhythmia the pulse rate increases with each inspiration and decreases with each expiration. This is normal. Sometimes ectopic beats occur regularly (e.g. every third beat).[5]

Character and volume

The character and volume of the pulse are better assessed from palpation of the brachial or carotid arteries. However, the

---

5 This is called a *trigeminal* rhythm.

collapsing (bounding) pulse of aortic regurgitation may be apparent at the wrist (see Table 4.3).

The blood pressure

The systolic blood pressure is the peak pressure that occurs in the artery following ventricular systole, and the diastolic blood pressure is the level to which the arterial blood pressure falls during ventricular diastole.

High blood pressure

The risk of adverse outcome increases as the blood pressure rises above normal. **Malignant hypertension** is marked hypertension (usually the diastolic is >120 mmHg) with changes on fundoscopy (haemorrhages, exudates and papilloedema; see p. 233).

Postural blood pressure

The blood pressure should be taken routinely with the patient lying and standing (or sitting). A fall of more than 15 mmHg in systolic blood pressure or 10 mmHg in diastolic blood pressure on standing is abnormal and is called **postural hypotension**. It may not be associated with symptoms.

Changes with respiration: pulsus paradoxus

A **fall in systolic blood** pressure of up to 10 mmHg occurs normally during inspiration. Exaggeration of this response—a fall of more than 10 mmHg—is an important sign of pericardial tamponade (rapid accumulation of fluid in the pericardial space) or severe asthma.

- It is detected by lowering the cuff pressure slowly from a level above the systolic pressure. The expiratory systolic blood pressure will be detected when Korotkoff I (KI) sounds are heard intermittently. As the cuff pressure is lowered there will be a point when KI sounds are heard throughout the respiratory cycle.
- The difference between these two readings gives the level of pulsus paradoxus.

The face

1. Look for **xanthelasma**: these intracutaneous yellow cholesterol deposits around the eyes are relatively common (see Fig 4.6a). They may be a normal variant or may indicate hyperlipidaemia.

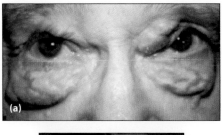

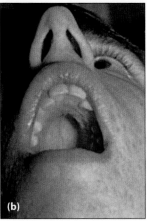

Figure 4.6   Examining the face. **(a)** Xanthelasma. (McDonald FS, ed. *Mayo Clinic Images in Internal Medicine*, with permission. © Mayo Clinic Scientific Press and CRC Press.) **(b)** High arched palate (Marfan's syndrome). (Forbes CD, Jackson WF. *Color Atlas and Text of Clinical Medicine*. Elsevier; 2003.)

2. In the mouth, use a torch to see if there is a **high arched palate** (see Fig 4.6b). This occurs in *Marfan's syndrome*, a condition that is associated with congenital heart disease, including aortic regurgitation secondary to aortic dilation, and also mitral regurgitation due to mitral valve prolapse.

3. Look for **diseased teeth** as they can be a source of organisms responsible for infective endocarditis.

4. Look at the tongue and lips for **central cyanosis**, which refers to a blue discolouration from an abnormal amount of deoxygenated haemoglobin in parts of the body with a good circulation.

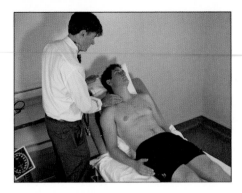

Figure 4.7 Feeling the carotid pulse (not too hard and only one side at a time).

The neck

Useful information about cardiac function is available in most necks. Arterial (carotid) and venous (jugular) pulsations should be examined.

Carotid arteries

The carotid pulse can be felt medial to the sternocleidomastoid muscle by applying slight posterior and medial pressure with the middle and forefingers (see Fig 4.7). Evaluation of the **amplitude**, **character** and **volume** of the pulse is used to help in the diagnosis of various underlying cardiac diseases and in assessing their severity (see Table 4.3).

Jugular venous pressure

The internal jugular vein runs a direct course to the right atrium (see Fig 4.8). By convention, the sternal angle is taken as the zero point, and the maximum height of pulsations in the internal jugular vein, which are visible above this level when the patient is at 45°, can be measured in centimetres.

The **jugular venous pulsation can be distinguished from the arterial pulse:**

- the JVP is visible but not palpable
- moves on respiration—normally, the JVP decreases on inspiration
- has a complex wave form, usually seen to flicker twice with each cardiac cycle (if the patient is in sinus rhythm)
- is at first obliterated and then filled from above when light pressure is applied at the base of the neck.

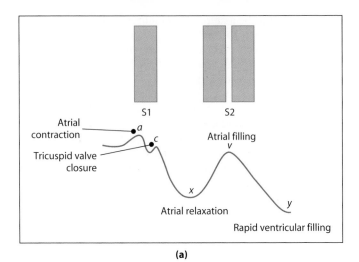

(a)

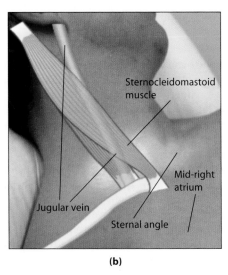

(b)

Figure 4.8   **(a)** Jugular venous pulsation and its relationship to the first (S1) and second (S2) heart sounds (Talley N, O'Connor S. *Clinical Examination 7e.* Elsevier; 2014, Figure 5.24.) **(b)** The anatomy of the neck showing the relative positions of the main vascular structures, clavicle and sternocleidomastoid muscle. (Adapted from Douglas G, Nicol F, Robertson C. *Macleod's Clinical Examination 11e.* Elsevier; 2005.)

The JVP must be assessed for **height** and **character**:

- When the JVP is more than 3 cm above the zero point, the right heart filling pressure is raised. This is a sign of right ventricular failure or volume overload.
- There are two positive waves in the normal JVP. The first is called the **a wave** and coincides with right atrial systole. It is due to atrial contraction. The a wave also coincides with the first heart sound and precedes the carotid pulsation. The second impulse is called the **v wave** and is due to atrial filling in the period when the tricuspid valve remains closed during ventricular systole (see Fig 4.8).

JVP rises on inspiration

Any condition in which right ventricular filling is limited (e.g. constrictive pericarditis, cardiac tamponade or right ventricular infarction) can cause elevation of the venous pressure, which is more marked on inspiration when venous return to the heart increases. This rise in the JVP on inspiration, called *Kussmaul's sign*, is the opposite of what normally happens. This sign is best elicited with the patient sitting up at 90° and breathing quietly through the mouth.

Cannon a waves occur when the right atrium contracts against the closed tricuspid valve (i.e. the ventricles and atria have contracted at the same time). This is usually a result of cardiac electrical abnormalities which have resulted in dissociation of atrial and ventricular contraction (e.g. complete heart block).

Large v waves occur in tricuspid regurgitation. Some of the right ventricular output regurgitates through the leaking tricuspid valve and wells up into the superior vena cava and from there into the jugular vein.

The **abdominojugular reflux test** can be performed as a test of right ventricular failure if the JVP is not raised. The examiner applies steady pressure over the right upper or middle abdomen for 10 seconds. There may be a brief rise in the JVP to over 4 cm. If this is sustained for the duration of the compression, the test is positive. This is a reliable sign of right ventricular failure.

THE PRAECORDIUM

The praecordium should be examined anteriorly by inspection, palpation and auscultation.

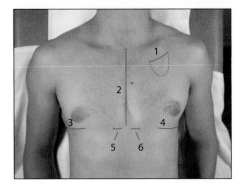

Figure 4.9 Model with lines showing surgical and pacemaker scars. 1 = pacemaker scar, 2 = median sternotomy scar, 3 + 4 = right and left lateral thoractomy scars, 5 + 6 = surgical drain scars.

Inspection
You will be **looking for:**

- chest wall scars
- apex beat (visible contraction of the left ventricle during systole).

1. Inspect first for **scars** and **lumps**. Previous cardiac operations will have left scars on the chest wall.
   - Coronary artery and valve surgery are usually performed through a median sternotomy incision and a scar will be visible extending from just below the suprasternal notch to the xiphisternum.
   - Another surgical 'abnormality' is a **pacemaker box**. These are usually under the right or left pectoral muscle, are usually easily palpable and are obviously metallic (see Fig 4.9).
2. The **apex beat** may be visible as a flickering movement of a small area (about 2 cm) of the skin of the chest wall between two ribs. It is caused by the twisting or wringing movement that occurs with ventricular systole (contraction). Its normal position is in the fifth left intercostal space 1 cm medial to the midclavicular line (see Fig 4.10).

Palpation
You will be trying to **feel** for:

- apex beat
- thrills (palpable murmurs)
- other impulses.

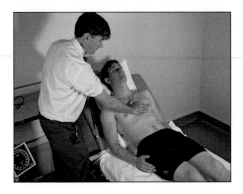

Figure 4.10   Finding the apex beat.

1. Count down the number of interspaces (use the tips of your fingers) to where the **apex beat** is palpable (see Fig 4.10).[6] The first palpable rib interspace is the second. The position of the apex beat is defined as the most lateral and inferior point at which the palpating fingers are raised with each systole. An apex beat displaced laterally or inferiorly, or both, usually indicates enlargement of the heart, but may occasionally be due to chest wall deformity, or pleural or pulmonary disease. The normal apex beat gently lifts the palpating fingers. Try to decide whether the apex beat is normal or abnormal.
   - The **dyskinetic** apex beat feels uncoordinated and large. It is usually due to left ventricular dysfunction (e.g. previous anterior myocardial infarction or dilated cardiomyopathy).
   - The **volume loaded** (hyperkinetic or diastolic overloaded) apex beat is a coordinated impulse felt over a larger area than normal in the praecordium and is usually the result of left ventricular dilation (e.g. due to aortic regurgitation).
   - The **pressure loaded** (hyperdynamic or systolic overloaded) apex beat is a forceful and sustained impulse. This occurs with aortic stenosis or hypertension.

---

6 In about 50% of people, the apex beat is not palpable. This is most often due to a thick chest wall, emphysema, pericardial effusion, shock (or death) and very rarely to dextrocardia (where there is inversion of the heart and great vessels). The apex beat will be palpable to the right of the sternum in many cases of dextrocardia.

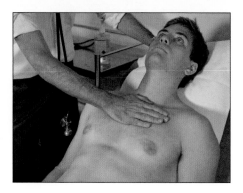

Figure 4.11   Palpating the base of the heart for palpable murmurs (thrills)—push firmly.

2. Turbulent blood flow, which is what causes cardiac murmurs on auscultation, may sometimes be palpable. These palpable murmurs are called **thrills**. The praecordium should be systematically palpated for thrills with the flat of the hand (palm side), first over the apex and left sternal edge, and then over the base of the heart (this is the upper part of the chest and includes the aortic and pulmonary areas; see Fig 4.11).

    Apical thrills can be more easily felt with the patient rolled over to the left side (the left lateral position) as this brings the apex closer to the chest wall. Thrills may also be palpable over the **base of the heart**. These may be maximal over the pulmonary or aortic areas, depending on the underlying cause, and are best felt with the patient sitting up, leaning forwards and in full expiration. In this position the base of the heart is moved closer to the chest wall.

    - A thrill that coincides in time with the apex beat is called a **systolic thrill**.
    - A thrill that does not coincide with the apex beat is called a **diastolic thrill**.

    The presence of a thrill usually means there is a significant abnormality of the heart and that the associated murmur is not an **innocent** (normal variation) murmur.

3. Feel also for a **parasternal impulse**. The heel of the hand is rested just to the left of the sternum with the fingers lifted slightly off the chest. In cases of right ventricular enlargement or severe left atrial enlargement, where the right ventricle is pushed anteriorly, the heel of the hand is lifted off the chest wall with each systole.

   Palpation with the fingers over the pulmonary area (second left intercostal space) may reveal the *palpable tap of pulmonary valve closure* in cases of pulmonary hypertension.

Auscultation

You will be **listening** in each area of the heart for:

- heart sounds (first and second)
- extra heart sounds (third and fourth)
- additional sounds (e.g. snaps, clicks or prosthetic heart sounds)
- murmurs (which you will need to time, then determine the area of greatest intensity, assess loudness and pitch, and, if indicated, perform dynamic manoeuvres)
- rubs.

1. Auscultation of the heart traditionally begins in the mitral area (see Fig 4.3) with the bell of the stethoscope. This better amplifies low-pitched sounds, such as the murmur of mitral stenosis (see Fig 4.12). It must be applied lightly to the chest wall.

2. Next listen in the mitral area with the diaphragm of the stethoscope, which best reproduces higher-pitched sounds, such as the systolic murmur of mitral regurgitation. Some newer stethoscopes reproduce the effect of the bell when the auscultator presses the diaphragm lightly on the chest and of the diaphragm when it is applied more firmly.[7] Now place the stethoscope in the tricuspid area (fifth left intercostal space) and listen. Next inch up the left sternal edge to the pulmonary (second left intercostal space) and aortic (second right intercostal space) areas, listening carefully in each position with the diaphragm.

---

7 This is convenient but deprives the clinician of a rotating stethoscope head to manipulate at times of worry.

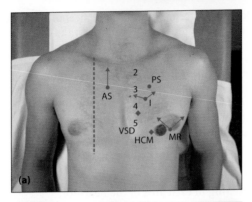

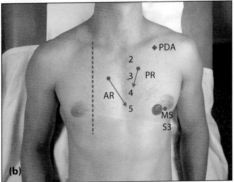

(2–5 refer to intercostal spaces; dotted line = midclavicular line)

(a) Systolic murmurs:

AS = aortic stenosis
MR = mitral regurgitation
HCM = hypertrophic cardiomyopathy
PS = pulmonary stenosis
VSD = ventricular septal defect
I = innocent

(b) Diastolic murmurs and sounds:

AR = aortic regurgitation
MS = mitral stenosis
S3 = third heart sound
PR = pulmonary regurgitation
PDA = patent ductus arteriosus (continuous murmur)

Figure 4.12 Radiation and sites of maximum intensity of heart sounds and murmurs. The midclavicular line (on the right) is shown for illustrative purposes.

3. **Heart sounds**. Auscultation of the normal heart reveals two sounds called, not surprisingly, the **first** and **second heart sounds**:

   • The **first heart sound (S1)** has two components: mitral and tricuspid valve closure. Mitral valve closure occurs slightly before that of the tricuspid valve, but usually only one sound is audible. The first heart sound indicates the beginning of ventricular contraction (systole); ventricular relaxation is called diastole.

   • The **second heart sound (S2)** at the apex is generally softer, shorter and higher pitched than the first (see Fig 4.13). It marks the end of systole and is made up of sounds from aortic and pulmonary valve closures. In normal cases, because of lower pressure in the pulmonary circulation compared with the aorta, closure of the pulmonary valve is later than that of the aortic valve. These components are usually sufficiently separated in time so that **splitting** of the second heart sound is audible and is best appreciated in the pulmonary area and along the left sternal edge.

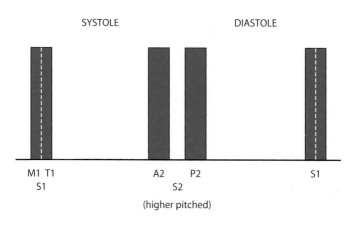

S1 = first heart sound; S2 = second heart sound;
M1 = mitral component of S1; T1 = tricuspid component of S1;
A2 = aortic component of S2; P2 = pulmonary component of S2.

Figure 4.13 Normal heart sounds.

Pulmonary valve closure is further delayed with inspiration because of increased venous return to the right ventricle, and thus splitting of the second heart sound is wider on inspiration. The second heart sound marks the beginning of diastole, which is usually longer than systole.

It can be difficult to decide which heart sound is which. Palpation of the carotid pulsation in the neck will indicate the timing of systole and enable the heart sounds to be distinguished more easily.

T&O'C examination hint box: Abnormalities of the heart sounds

Alterations in intensity
- S1 is **loud** when the mitral or tricuspid valve cusps remain widely open at the end of diastole and shut forcefully with the onset of ventricular systole (see Fig 4.14). This occurs in mitral stenosis where the valve orifice has become narrowed, usually as a result of scarring of the leaflets from rheumatic fever.
- **Soft** S1 can be due to failure of the leaflets to coapt normally (as in mitral regurgitation, where blood leaks back from the left ventricle into the left atrium during systole—this used to be called mitral incompetence or insufficiency).
- S2 may have a **loud aortic component (A2)** in patients with systemic hypertension.
- The **pulmonary component of the second heart sound (P2)** is loud in pulmonary hypertension, where the valve closure may be forceful because of the high pulmonary pressure.
- A **soft A2** will be found when the aortic valve is calcified and leaflet movement is reduced, and in aortic regurgitation when the leaflets cannot coapt.

Splitting (see Fig 4.14)
- Splitting of S1 is not usually detectable clinically; however, when it occurs it is most often due to complete right bundle branch block (a cardiac conduction abnormality).
- **Increased normal splitting** (wider on inspiration) of S2 occurs when there is any delay in right ventricular emptying, as in right bundle branch block (delayed right ventricular depolarisation) or pulmonary stenosis (delayed right ventricular ejection).
- In the case of **fixed splitting** the normal respiratory variation is absent and splitting tends to be wide. This is caused by an atrial septal defect where equalisation of volume loads between the two atria occurs through the defect.

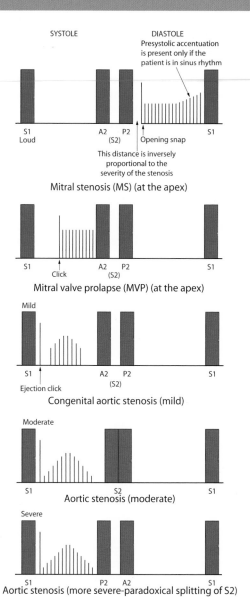

Figure 4.14 Heart sounds: snaps, clicks and splitting.

4. **Extra heart sounds**.
   - The **third heart sound (S3)** is a low-pitched, mid-diastolic sound that is best appreciated by listening for the characteristic triple cadence of the cardiac rhythm. It has been likened (not unreasonably) to the sound of a galloping horse and is often called a gallop rhythm. It can be physiological in pregnancy; otherwise, it is an important sign of left ventricular failure but may also occur in aortic regurgitation or mitral regurgitation.
   - The **fourth heart sound (S4)** is a late diastolic sound that is slightly more high-pitched than S3. Again, this is responsible for the impression of a triple (gallop) rhythm. It is never physiological and is most often due to systemic hypertension. It cannot be present if the patient has atrial fibrillation because it corresponds to atrial systole.

T&O'C examination essentials

Signs of cardiac failure (in approximate order of helpfulness)

Right ventricular failure
Right ventricular third heart sound
Elevated jugular venous pressure
Signs of tricuspid regurgitation—large v waves, pulsatile liver
Peripheral oedema
Ascites

Left ventricular failure
Third heart sound
Displaced and dyskinetic apex beat
Bilateral basal inspiratory crackles (medium or coarse)
Dyspnoea and especially orthopnoea (a symptom and a sign)
Pleural effusion (left or bilateral)

---

5. **Additional sounds**.
   - An **opening snap** is a high-pitched sound that occurs in mitral stenosis at a variable distance after S2 (see Fig 4.14). It is due to the sudden opening of the mitral valve and is followed by the diastolic murmur of mitral stenosis. It is best heard at the lower left sternal edge with the diaphragm of the stethoscope.

- A **systolic ejection click** is an early systolic, high-pitched sound heard over the aortic or pulmonary area, which may occur in cases of congenital aortic or pulmonary stenosis where the valve remains mobile; it is followed by the systolic ejection murmur of aortic or pulmonary stenosis.
- A **non-ejection systolic click** is a high-pitched sound heard during systole and is best appreciated at the mitral area. It is a common finding. It may be followed by a systolic murmur. The click may be due to prolapse of one or both redundant mitral valve leaflets during systole.
- Mechanical prosthetic heart valves produce characteristic **crisp metallic sounds**. Older caged-ball valves[8] make much more noise than modern leaflet valves.

T&O'C examination hint box

Use of the term 'opening snap' implies the diagnosis of mitral stenosis—only use the term if you have made that diagnosis (classical signs include a loud S1 and a low-pitched rumbling diastolic murmur over the mitral area).

6. **Murmurs of the heart**.

   The correct diagnosis of a murmur depends on the synthesis of findings made at the praecordium (apex beat, thrills etc), the noise itself and the peripheral signs.

   - *Timing* (see Table 4.4). **Systolic murmurs** (which occur during ventricular systole) may be pansystolic, ejection systolic or late systolic.
     - The **pansystolic murmur** extends throughout systole, beginning with S1 and going right up to S2. Causes of pansystolic murmurs include mitral regurgitation, tricuspid regurgitation and ventricular septal defect.
     - An **ejection systolic** murmur does not begin right at S1; its intensity is greatest in mid-systole or later and

---

8 Starr-Edwards caged-ball valves can be heard across a crowded room. Most patients have become used to the sound and say they are only worried if the noise stops.

TABLE 4.4   Cardiac murmurs

Timing	Lesion	Maximum intensity
SYSTOLIC		
Pansystolic	Mitral regurgitation	Apex
	Tricuspid regurgitation	Lower left sternal edge
	Ventricular septal defect	Lower left sternal edge
Ejection systolic	Aortic stenosis	Base (aortic area)
	Pulmonary stenosis	Base (pulmonary area)
	Hypertrophic cardiomyopathy[9]	Lower left sternal edge
	Pulmonary flow murmur of an atrial septal defect	Pulmonary area
Late systolic	Mitral valve prolapse	Apex
	Papillary muscle dysfunction (due usually to ischaemia or hypertrophic cardiomyopathy)	Apex
DIASTOLIC		
Early diastolic	Aortic regurgitation	Lower left sternal edge
	Pulmonary regurgitation	Left sternal edge
Mid-diastolic	Mitral stenosis	Apex
	Tricuspid stenosis	Right lower sternal edge
Presystolic	Mitral stenosis	Apex
	Tricuspid stenosis	Right lower sternal edge
	Atrial myxoma	Apex

9 Genetic cardiac muscle disease causing left ventricular hypertrophy and outflow obstruction leading to a systolic murmur.

TABLE 4.4 Cardiac murmurs *continued*

Timing	Lesion	Maximum intensity
DIASTOLIC *continued*		
Continuous	Patent ductus arteriosus	Below left clavicle
	Arteriovenous fistula (coronary artery, pulmonary, systemic)	Left sternal edge
	Aorto-pulmonary connection	Left sternal edge
	Venous hum (abolished by ipsilateral internal jugular vein compression)	Supraclavicular fossa
	Rupture of sinus of Valsalva into right ventricle or atrium	Left sternal edge

Note: The combined murmurs of aortic stenosis and aortic regurgitation, or mitral stenosis and mitral regurgitation, may sound as if they fill the entire cardiac cycle but they are not continuous murmurs by definition.

wanes again late in systole. This is described as a crescendo–decrescendo murmur. These murmurs are usually caused by turbulent flow through the aortic or pulmonary valve orifices or by greatly increased flow through a normal-sized orifice or outflow tract.

- If a murmur is **late systolic**, one is able to distinguish a gap between S1 and the murmur, which then continues right up to S2. This is typical of mitral valve prolapse or papillary muscle dysfunction.

- **Diastolic murmurs** occur during ventricular diastole.
  - The **early diastolic murmur** begins immediately with S2 and has a decrescendo quality (i.e. it is loudest at the beginning and extends for a variable distance into diastole). These early diastolic murmurs are typically high-pitched and are due to

regurgitation through a leaking aortic or (less commonly) pulmonary valve.

- **Mid-diastolic murmurs** begin later in diastole and may be short or extend right up to S1. They have a much lower-pitched quality than early diastolic murmurs. They are due to impaired flow during ventricular filling and can be caused by mitral stenosis where the valve is narrowed.
- **Presystolic murmurs** may be heard when atrial systole increases blood flow across the valve just before S1. They are an extension of the mid-diastolic murmurs of mitral stenosis and are absent in patients who are in atrial fibrillation (because atrial systole is lost).

- **Continuous murmurs** extend throughout systole and diastole. They are produced when a communication exists between two parts of the circulation with a permanent pressure gradient so that blood flow occurs continuously (e.g. patent [persistent] ductus arteriosus). They should be distinguished from combined systolic and diastolic murmurs (due, for example, to aortic stenosis and aortic regurgitation).
- *Area of greatest intensity and radiation.* Unfortunately the place on the praecordium where a murmur is loudest is not a very reliable guide to its origin.
  - For example, the murmur of mitral regurgitation, although clearly audible at the apex, may be heard widely over the praecordium and even right up into the aortic area or over the back.
  - Radiation of an ejection systolic murmur up into the carotid arteries suggests that this arises from the aortic valve.
  - Radiation of a systolic murmur to the axilla suggests mitral regurgitation.
  - The murmur of a ventricular septal defect is loudest in the right parasternal area and is not well heard at the base of the heart or at the apex. This helps distinguish it from the murmurs of aortic stenosis and mitral regurgitation, respectively.
- *Loudness and pitch.* The loudness of the murmur may not be helpful in deciding the severity of the valve

lesion. Harshness is perhaps a better guide. Changes in the loudness, however, are very important. Murmurs are usually graded according to loudness. Cardiologists often use a classification with six grades; most murmurs are grade 2 or 3:

- **grade 1/6:** very soft and only audible in ideal listening conditions (may only be audible if told it is present)[10]
- **grade 2/6:** soft, but can be detected almost immediately by an experienced auscultator
- **grade 3/6:** moderate; there is no thrill
- **grade 4/6:** loud; thrill just palpable
- **grade 5/6:** very loud; thrill easily palpable
- **grade 6/6:** very, very loud (and very uncommon); can be heard even without placing the stethoscope on the chest.

- *Dynamic manoeuvres.*
  - **Respiration**. Listen to the murmur as the patient breathes deeply in and out. Murmurs that arise on the right side of the heart tend to be louder during inspiration when increased venous return increases blood flow to the right side of the heart.
  - **Exercise**. If mitral stenosis is suspected but the diastolic murmur is difficult to hear, it is helpful to exercise the patient by getting him or her to sit up and down a number of times. Get the patient to then lie quickly on the left side and listen at the apex with the bell.

7. **Rubs.**
   - A **pericardial friction rub** is a superficial scratching sound; there may be up to three distinct components occurring at any time during the cardiac cycle. They are not confined to systole or diastole. A rub is caused by movement of inflamed pericardial surfaces. The sound can vary with respiration and posture; it is often louder when the patient is sitting up and breathing out. It tends to come and go.

---

10 Cannot be heard by medical students or new cardiologists who rely on their echo machine almost entirely.

THE BACK

Percussion and auscultation of the lung bases (see Ch 5) are also part of the cardiovascular examination. Signs of cardiac failure may be detected in the lungs; in particular, late or pan-inspiratory crackles or a pleural effusion (usually left-sided) may be present. Remember that basal crackles are common and not always due to cardiac failure. While the patient is sitting up, feel for *pitting oedema of the sacrum* (see below), which occurs in severe right heart failure, especially in patients who have been in bed.

THE ABDOMEN

Lay the patient down flat (on one pillow) and examine the abdomen (see Ch 6).

- The liver may become enlarged and tender due to hepatic venous congestion in patients with right ventricular failure.
- This may be accompanied by ascites (peritoneal fluid) in severe cases.
- A pulsatile liver is a reliable sign of tricuspid regurgitation.
- Splenomegaly may be present when a patient has infective endocarditis.

THE LEGS

1. Palpate the peripheral pulses.
   - Examine both femoral arteries (found by feeling in the inguinal crease midway between the anterior superior iliac spine and the pubic tubercle) (see Fig 4.15).
   - Examine the arteries of the legs on both sides (see Fig 4.16): the popliteal (behind the knee), posterior tibial (under the medial malleolus) and dorsalis pedis (on the forefoot—the dorsalis pedis pulse is congenitally absent in about 2% of patients).
2. Inspect for oedema and signs of arterial and venous disease.
   - Palpate the distal shaft of the tibia for oedema by compressing the area gently for at least 15 seconds with the thumb. If **pitting oedema** is present, a little pit will appear in the shape of the examiner's thumb and refill only gradually.

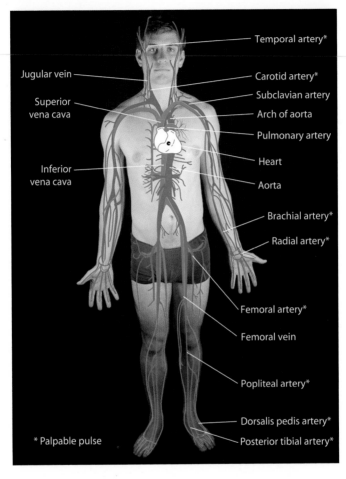

Temporal artery*
Jugular vein
Carotid artery*
Subclavian artery
Superior vena cava
Arch of aorta
Pulmonary artery
Heart
Inferior vena cava
Aorta
Brachial artery*
Radial artery*
Femoral artery*
Femoral vein
Popliteal artery*
Dorsalis pedis artery*
* Palpable pulse
Posterior tibial artery*

Figure 4.15   The palpable arteries (pulses) and the venous system.

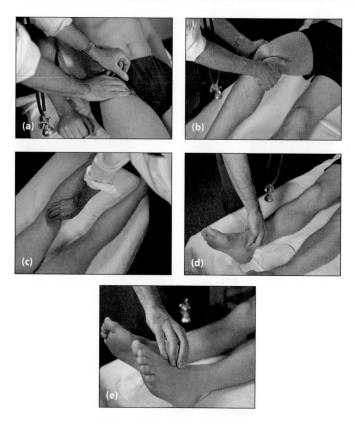

Figure 4.16 Sites of the peripheral pulses. **(a)** The femoral pulse is felt just below the inguinal ligament midway between the anterior superior iliac crest and the symphysis pubis. **(b)** To examine the popliteal artery, the leg is flexed to relax the hamstrings, and firm compression is applied against the lower end of the tibia. **(c)** The popliteal pulse can often be more easily felt when the patient is prone. **(d)** The posterior tibial artery is felt just behind the tip of the medial malleolus. **(e)** The dorsalis pedis is felt at the proximal end of the first intermetatarsal space.

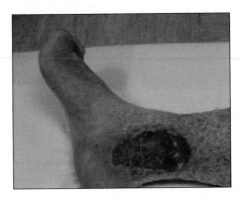

Figure 4.17   Venous ulcers are typically located at the medial aspect of the leg in the supramalleolar area. Their size and ulcer-bed condition are variable depending on ulcer duration and treatment. The periwound skin can be brown in colour and is usually hard because of dermatosclerosis typical of venous insufficiency. Scaling is another typical feature of venous ulcers. (Mosti G. Compression and venous surgery for venous leg ulcers. *Clinics in Plastic Surgery* 2012, 39(3): 269–280. © 2012, Figure 1.)

TABLE 4.5 Leg ulcers: clinical clues		
Venus ulcer	Arterial ulcer	Neuropathic ulcer (e.g. diabetic neuropathy)
Irregular margin Pale surrounding new skin Pink base Skin warm Pulses normal	Regular margin 'Punched out' appearance Skin cold No peripheral pulses	Painless Loss of skin sensation Skin warm Pulses normal

- Leg ulcers (which are typically on the medial side of the lower third of the leg above the medial malleolus when due to venous disease; see Fig 4.17 and Table 4.5) and varicose veins should be noted.
- This type of venous disease is often associated with venous staining of the skin. Haemosiderin deposited in

the skin as a result of increased venous pressure causes a blue-grey discolouration.

> **T&O'C examination hint box**
>
> If pitting oedema of the lower limbs makes palpation of the pedal pulses difficult, gentle pressure over the area for 10–15 seconds will temporarily displace fluid and assist.

- If varicose veins are present, the site of **venous valvular incompetence** should be determined. Examine for long saphenous incompetence as follows:
    - **Cough impulse test**. After standing the patient up, palpate just below the fossa ovalis (where the vein passes to join the femoral vein), which is 3 cm below and 3 cm lateral to the pubic tubercle, and ask the patient to cough. Feel for an impulse (thrill). Look also for a **saphena varix** (dilation of the vein that produces a swelling in the fossa ovalis, which, unlike a femoral hernia, disappears when the patient lies down).
    - **Trendelenberg test**. After lying the patient down, elevate the (patient's) leg to empty the veins. Then compress the upper end of the vein in the groin with your hand and stand the patient up; normally, if little or no filling occurs until the groin pressure is released, sapheno-femoral valve incompetence is present and the test is positive. If filling occurs before the pressure is released, incompetent veins are in the thigh or calf.
- The presence of calf pain at rest should suggest the possibility of **deep venous thrombosis**. Examine for swelling of the affected calf and dilated superficial veins. Tenderness and warmth may be present on palpation. These signs have, unfortunately, not been shown to be sensitive or specific for this condition.

T&O'C examination hint box 4.1: How to examine the patient with chest pain

1. Does the patient look unwell (breathless, cyanosed or sweaty)? Is the pain present now? Sweating and an appearance of anxiety can be associated with myocardial infarction or pulmonary embolism.
2. Measure the blood pressure. Low blood pressure can occur in cardiogenic shock from a large myocardial infarction or pulmonary embolism.
3. Take the pulse. Tachycardia suggests pain or pulmonary embolism.
4. If the pain extends to the back, measure the blood pressure in each arm. Aortic dissection can affect the left subclavian artery and reduce blood pressure on that side.
5. Examine the chest for signs of pneumonia, pleurisy or heart failure.
6. Examine the heart. Most patients with infarction have few signs, but a third heart sound may be a sign of a large infarct. Aortic stenosis can cause exertional chest pain.
7. If the pain is pleuritic, sit the patient up, leaning forwards, to listen for a pericardial rub.

T&O'C examination hint box 4.2: How to examine the patient with palpitations

(The examination is often normal.)
1. Take the pulse.
2. Examine the cardiovascular system, looking for signs of mitral valve disease (AF or flutter) or heart failure (VT).
3. Look for signs of thyrotoxicosis.

T&O'C examination hint box 4.3: How to examine the patient with ankle oedema

1. Look at the legs: how far does the swelling extend (e.g. to knees, thighs, genitals or even the abdominal wall)?
2. Look for varicose veins.
3. Look for venous ulceration or staining.
4. Press over the end of the tibia (not too hard) and look for pitting. Lymphoedema does not pit.
5. Look for joint problems or infection in the legs.
6. Examine the heart for signs of heart failure—specifically for a raised JVP, big v waves and a pulsatile liver (all signs of right heart failure).
7. Look for signs of chronic lung disease.

The cardiovascular examination OSCE: hints panel

This OSCE is usually centred around the diagnosis of common cardiac murmurs, signs of heart failure or peripheral vascular disease. The examiner will usually direct you to a region to be examined.

Always introduce yourself to the patient first and ask permission to perform an examination. Then wash your hands. Try to synthesise the findings as you go along.

1. This patient has been breathless on exertion and has a murmur. Please examine his praecordium.
   (a) Ask the patient to uncover his chest and stand back for a moment to look for breathlessness at rest, and cyanosis.
   (b) Look at the patient's chest for surgical scars or deformity. Look for the apex beat.
   (c) Feel for the apex beat, thrills and a parasternal impulse.
   (d) Listen with the bell and then the diaphragm at the apex. Listen with the diaphragm at the left sternal edge and at the base of the heart.
   (e) Sit the patient up and listen at the left sternal edge and at the base with the patient in deep expiration.
   (f) Listen over the carotids.
   (g) If you are confident of the diagnosis, tell the examiner; for example, 'I think this patient has aortic stenosis of moderate severity.' Then describe the physical findings. If you are unsure, describe the abnormal findings before committing to any diagnosis.
2. This woman has been breathless on exertion and wakes breathless at night. Please examine her.
   (a) Ask the patient to undress if necessary but leave a towel or part of a gown across her breasts.
   (b) Stand back to look for obvious breathlessness due to cardiac failure.
   (c) Look for cyanosis and clubbing, and take the pulse and blood pressure.
   (d) Look at the jugular venous pressure.
   (e) Look at the praecordium for the apex beat, scars etc.
   (f) Make a careful attempt to find and assess the apex beat. Feel for thrills and a parasternal impulse.
   (g) Auscultate for murmurs and a gallop rhythm.
   (h) Examine the chest posteriorly and look for peripheral oedema.
   (i) Synthesise and present your findings.
3. This man is a smoker and has pains in his calves when he walks. Please examine his legs.
   (a) Ask the patient to uncover his legs to at least the mid thighs.
   (b) Stand back for a general inspection; note dyspnoea, cyanosis and nicotine staining of the fingers.

     (c) Look at the legs for missing toes. Note cyanosis, hair loss over the lower legs or feet, and skin and calf muscle atrophy.

     (d) Examine the peripheral pulses, starting with the feet and working back to the femorals if the distal pulses are reduced or absent.

     (e) Look for the scars of previous peripheral bypass operations. These are usually seen extending longitudinally across the femoral artery.

     (f) Examine the abdomen (aortic aneurysm), then take the blood pressure.

     (g) Synthesise and present your findings.

4. This man has swelling of his ankles. Please examine his legs.

     (a) Ask the patient to uncover his legs, using a towel to cover his groin. Lay him flat if possible.

     (b) Stand back to look for peripheral oedema, and note its extent, abdominal distension (ascites), dyspnoea and signs of chronic lung disease (p. 115).

     (c) Examine for pitting oedema and establish its upper level. Remember that it may involve the genitals and abdominal wall if severe.

     (d) Look for varicose veins.

     (e) Examine the abdomen for ascites (p. 157), and feel the liver for enlargement and for signs of tricuspid regurgitation (liver pulsatile).

     (f) Palpate for sacral oedema.

     (g) Examine the heart and lungs.

     (h) Synthesise and present your findings.

5. This man has developed central chest pain of sudden onset. Please examine him.

     (a) Examine all relevant systems to narrow the differential diagnosis.

        (i) Check for radio-radial delay (aortic dissection).

        (ii) Examine the patient's pulses for arrhythmias.

        (iii) Take the patient's blood pressure.

        (iv) Look for signs of cardiac failure: JVP, oedema.

        (v) Auscultate the heart for a gallop rhythm (heart failure) and a new murmur (e.g. papillary muscle rupture causing severe mitral regurgitation; signs of a ventricular septal defect post myocardial infarction).

        (vi) Examine the chest wall for tenderness (costochondritis), and assess for any mediastinal shift (tension pneumothorax).

        (vii) Palpate the abdomen for tenderness (referred pain).

        (viii) Examine the back (referred pain).

     (b) Synthesise and present your findings.

T&O'C examination essentials

The cardiovascular system

1. Ischaemic heart disease should be suspected from the history. When angina is stable, the pain or discomfort occurs with a predictable amount of exertion and is relieved by rest. A recent increase in the frequency or the occurrence of pain at rest suggests worsening (previously called unstable) angina.

2. Cardiac dyspnoea (i.e. breathlessness due to cardiac failure) is worse on exertion or when the patient lies flat (orthopnoea).

3. Ask about cardiac risk factors in any patient with suspected cardiac disease; for example, known high levels of cholesterol and triglycerides, smoking, hypertension, diabetes mellitus, family history of cardiac disease in first-degree relatives.

4. Pay particular attention when examining the cardiovascular system to the rate, rhythm and character of the pulse, the level of the blood pressure, elevation of the JVP, the position of the apex beat, and the presence of the heart sounds, any extra sounds or murmurs.

5. The position and timing of cardiac murmurs give important clues about the underlying valve lesion.

6. Remember the reliable signs of heart failure: displaced apex beat, S3, positive hepatojugular reflux test, raised JVP.

7. Important but less reliable signs of heart failure: lung crackles and peripheral oedema.

8. The diastolic murmur of aortic regurgitation is characteristic (high-pitched early diastolic murmur at the left sternal edge, increased by sitting up and holding breathing in expiration) and has high diagnostic utility.

The chest

Learn to see, learn to hear, learn to feel, learn to smell and know that by practice alone can you become experts.

Sir William Osler (1849–1919)

In this chapter, the symptoms and signs of lung disease are presented. The assessment begins with the history (concentrating in detail on the presenting symptoms). As usual, the examination begins with an assessment of the peripheral signs of lung disease and progresses to an examination of the chest, as set out below.

The respiratory system assessment sequence

1. Presenting symptoms (e.g. dyspnoea, cough, wheeze, fever)
2. Detailed questions about presenting symptoms (SOCRATES)
3. Questions about previous lung problems and respiratory risk factors (e.g. smoking, occupation, pets)
4. Examination for peripheral signs of respiratory disease
5. Examination of the chest
6. Provisional and differential diagnosis

The respiratory history

PRESENTING SYMPTOMS (see Box 5.1)

Cough and sputum

Cough is a common presenting respiratory symptom. Ask about the duration and whether:

- the cough is dry or productive (i.e. of sputum)
- it is associated with wheeze
- the patient is taking any medications.

Since the quality of the cough is important, ask the patient to describe the type of cough and to give a demonstration.

T&O'C examination essentials

Differential diagnosis of cough

1. A **cough of recent origin**, particularly if associated with fever and other symptoms of respiratory tract infection, may be due to acute bronchitis or pneumonia.
2. A **chronic cough associated with wheezing** may be due to asthma; sometimes asthma can present without wheeze.
3. An **irritating chronic dry cough** can result from the reflux of acid into the oesophagus or the use of certain antihypertensive drugs (angiotensin-converting enzyme [ACE] inhibitors).
4. A change in the **character** of a chronic cough may indicate the development of a new and serious underlying problem (e.g. infection or lung cancer).
5. A large volume of **purulent** (yellow or green) **sputum** suggests the diagnosis of bronchiectasis or lobar pneumonia.
6. **Foul-smelling, dark-coloured sputum** may indicate the presence of a lung abscess with anaerobic organisms.
7. **Pink frothy secretions** from the trachea, which occur in pulmonary oedema, should not be confused with sputum.
8. **Haemoptysis** (coughing up of blood) can be a sinister sign of lung disease and must always be investigated, because it may be due to carcinoma of the lung, pneumonia, tuberculosis, pulmonary infarction or bronchiectasis.

Box 5.1
The respiratory history: presenting symptoms

Major symptoms
Cough
Sputum
Haemoptysis
Dyspnoea (acute or chronic, progressive or paroxysmal)
Wheeze
Chest pain
Fever
Hoarseness

Dyspnoea

Ask about the timing of onset, severity and pattern of dyspnoea.

T&O'C examination hint box

- Patients with a history of *smoking* or *occupational dust exposure* often have a respiratory cause for dyspnoea.
- The presence of fever or a productive cough also points to a lung problem.
- If unrelated to position and associated with a wheeze and cough, then dyspnoea at night may be due to cold- or allergen-induced (e.g. house dust mite) bronchoconstriction.
- *Exertional dyspnoea* associated with a sensation of chest tightness may be a presentation of angina.

In three out of four cases the cause of dyspnoea can be diagnosed from the history.

Dyspnoea can be graded from I to IV (see Box 5.2). It may be more useful, however, to determine the amount of exertion that is actually needed to cause dyspnoea (i.e. the distance walked, or the number of steps climbed) or the patient's ability to perform daily tasks such as dressing and washing.

T&O'C examination hint box

Dyspnoea that is *worse when the patient lies flat* or that *wakes the patient from sleep* is more likely to be due to cardiac failure than lung disease.

> **Box 5.2**
> **Grading the severity of dyspnoea**
>
> - **Class I**—dyspnoea on heavy exertion
> - **Class II**—dyspnoea on moderate exertion
> - **Class III**—dyspnoea on minimal exertion
> - **Class IV**—dyspnoea at rest

> **Questions box 5.1** What to ask the patient complaining of breathlessness
>
> ❗ denotes a possible urgent or dangerous problem
> 1. How long have you been breathless?
> 2. Is it intermittent?
> 3. Is it getting worse?
> 4. Does it occur when you try to exercise?
> 5. How much exercise can you do before it occurs? Can you walk indefinitely on the flat/one flight of stairs?
> ❗ 6. Are you breathless at rest? On lying down? (Orthopnoea)
> 7. Are you wheezy? (Airway obstruction) Does the wheeze come and go?
> 8. Do you cough up sputum? If so, recently or for a long time? (Pneumonia vs bronchiectasis)
> 9. Have you had a high temperature?
> ❗ 10. Has the breathlessness come on suddenly? (Pulmonary embolism) Instantaneously? (Pneumothorax)
> 11. Have you worked with industrial gases or dusts? (Hypersensitivity pneumonitis, interstitial lung disease)
> ❗ 12. Is the breathlessness associated with a feeling of tightness in the chest? (Angina, aortic stenosis, HCM [hypertrophic cardiomyopathy])
> 13. Is the problem that you cannot get a satisfying breath? (Anxiety)

Wheeze

A number of conditions can cause a continuous whistling noise that is often louder during expiration (wheeze). These include asthma, chronic obstructive pulmonary disease (chronic obstructive airways disease), airway obstruction by a foreign body or tumour, and pulmonary oedema (severe cardiac failure).

Chest pain

Chest pain due to respiratory disease is characteristically *pleuritic* in nature (i.e. sharp and worse with deep inspiration and coughing). Thoracic muscle soreness is common when patients have an acute respiratory illness and cough.

Other presenting symptoms

- Patients may occasionally present with episodes of **fever at night** (e.g. tuberculosis and pneumonia) or **hoarseness** (e.g. laryngitis, vocal cord tumour or recurrent laryngeal nerve palsy).
- Patients with **obstructive sleep apnoea** (where airflow stops despite persistent respiratory efforts during sleep) typically present with daytime sleepiness (somnolence), chronic fatigue, morning headaches and personality disturbances. Very loud snoring may be reported by anyone within earshot.
- Some patients respond to anxiety by increasing the rate and depth of their breathing. This is called **hyperventilation**. The resultant alkalosis may result in paraesthesia of the fingers and around the mouth, light-headedness, chest pain and a feeling of impending collapse.
- **Anxiety** (e.g. during a panic attack) can also make patients feel that they need to take deep breaths or that they are unable to take a satisfying breath.

PAST HISTORY

Always ask about any previous respiratory illness (including pneumonia, tuberculosis and exacerbations of chronic bronchitis) or abnormalities of the chest X-ray or computed tomography (CT) scan that have been previously reported to the patient.

TREATMENT

Take a drug history:
- What drugs is the patient using?
- How often are these drugs taken? Are they inhaled or swallowed?

Almost every class of drug can produce lung toxicity. Examples include pulmonary embolism from use of the oral contraceptive pill, interstitial lung disease from cytotoxic agents, bronchospasm from beta-blockers or aspirin, and cough from ACE inhibitors.

OCCUPATIONAL HISTORY

Ask in some detail about:

- possible exposure to *dusts* in mines and factories (e.g. asbestos, coal, silica, iron oxide, tin oxide, cotton, beryllium, titanium oxide, silver, nitrogen dioxide or anhydrides)
- work or household exposure to *animals*, including birds (e.g. Q fever or psittacosis)
- exposure to *mouldy hay*, humidifiers or air-conditioners, which may also result in lung disease (e.g. hypersensitivity pneumonitis)
- exposure to spray painting and wood dusts, which may provoke *occupational asthma* that typically resolves on weekends or on holidays.

SOCIAL HISTORY

A smoking history (see Ch 1) must be taken as a routine. Find out who is at home as a support for the patient, especially if the respiratory disease has caused debilitating symptoms.

FAMILY HISTORY

There may be a family history of asthma, cystic fibrosis or emphysema. Alpha$_1$-antitrypsin deficiency, for example, is an inherited disease associated with a family history of the development of emphysema in young middle-age.

Examination anatomy

The examination of the lungs makes more sense when the basic anatomy and function of the lungs and airways are kept in mind (see Figs 5.1 and 5.2). Always try to picture the structures that lie beneath the area of the chest being examined.

Examining the chest

Examination of the chest should include a search for signs of lung disease (see Box 5.3), chest wall abnormalities and, if relevant, examination of the female breasts (see Ch 10). The patient should be undressed to the waist and, if well enough, should sit over the edge of the bed.

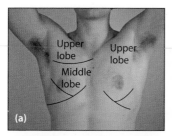
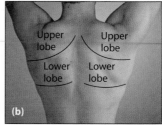
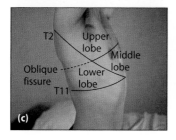
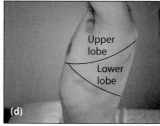

Figure 5.1 Lobes of the lung—surface markings. **(a)** Anterior.
(b) Posterior. **(c)** Right lateral. **(d)** Left lateral.

Box 5.3
The chest examination sequence

1. General appearance
2. Peripheral signs of lung disease
3. Assess the cough and look for the sputum mug
4. Examine the face
5. Feel the trachea
6. Test the forced expiratory time
7. Examine the chest:
   - inspection
   - palpation
   - percussion
   - auscultation
8. Examine the heart
9. Examine the abdomen

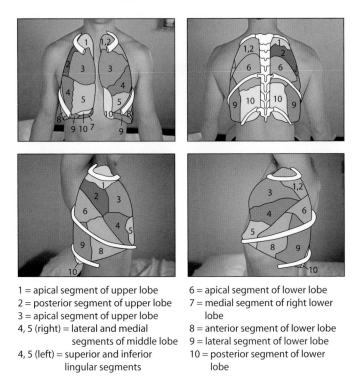

1 = apical segment of upper lobe
2 = posterior segment of upper lobe
3 = apical segment of upper lobe
4, 5 (right) = lateral and medial
        segments of middle lobe
4, 5 (left) = superior and inferior
        lingular segments

6 = apical segment of lower lobe
7 = medial segment of right lower
    lobe
8 = anterior segment of lower lobe
9 = lateral segment of lower lobe
10 = posterior segment of lower
     lobe

Figure 5.2 Surface markings of the segments of the lungs.

GENERAL APPEARANCE

In the ward, clinic or exam, note whether the patient looks well or unwell.

1. Does the patient appear unwell or in distress with the effort of breathing?
2. Look (and listen) for:
    * tachypnoea (a respiratory rate of more than 25 breaths per minute)
    * use of the accessory muscles of respiration during inspiration (sternocleidomastoids and scalene muscles; see Fig 5.3)
    * cyanosis

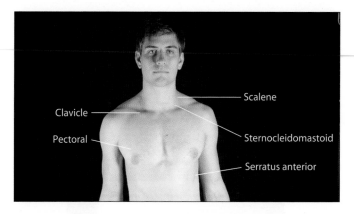

Figure 5.3   Use of the accessory muscles of respiration at rest (most reliably the scalene and sternocleidomastoid muscles) is a sign of respiratory distress.

- wheeze
- a spontaneous cough.

THE PERIPHERAL SIGNS OF LUNG DISEASE

The hands

Pick up the patient's right hand, then the left.

1. Look for **clubbing** (see Table 3.2). Respiratory causes of clubbing include carcinoma of the lung, chronic lung suppuration (e.g. pulmonary abscess, tuberculosis, bronchiectasis) and interstitial lung disease.

> **T&O'C examination essentials**
>
> Chronic obstructive pulmonary disease alone does *not* cause nail clubbing.

2. Look for **cigarette staining of the fingers** (actually caused by tar, because nicotine is colourless), more an indication of the way the patient holds the cigarette than of the number of cigarettes smoked.

3. Compression and infiltration by a peripheral lung tumour of a lower trunk of the brachial plexus result in **wasting** of the small muscles of the hands (see Fig 5.4).

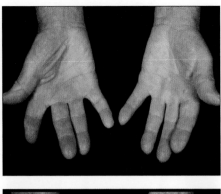
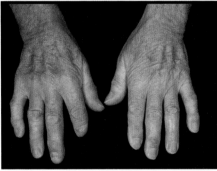

Figure 5.4 Wasting of the small muscles of the hands from lung cancer. (Perkin et al. *Atlas of Clinical Neurology 3e.* Copyright © 2011 by Saunders, an imprint of Elsevier Inc.)

The wrist and arm

Measure the pulse rate and blood pressure. Tachycardia and pulsus paradoxus are important signs of severe asthma.

Character of the cough

1. Ask the patient to cough several times.
   - Lack of the usual explosive beginning may indicate vocal cord paralysis (the 'bovine' cough).
   - A muffled, wheezy ineffective cough suggests chronic obstructive pulmonary disease.
   - A very loose, productive cough suggests excessive bronchial secretions due to chronic bronchitis, pneumonia or bronchiectasis.

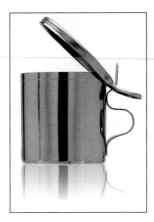

Figure 5.5   Sputum mug.

- A dry, irritating cough may occur with chest infection, asthma or carcinoma of the bronchus and less commonly with left ventricular failure or interstitial lung disease.
2. Impress your examiners and search for the **sputum** mug (see Fig 5.5) noting:
   - volume of sputum
   - type of sputum (purulent, mucoid or muco-purulent)
   - presence or absence of blood.
3. Obstruction of the larynx, trachea or large airways may cause **stridor**, a rasping or croaking noise loudest on inspiration. This can be due to a foreign body, a tumour, an infection (e.g. epiglottitis) or inflammation.

Hoarseness

Listen to the voice for **hoarseness**. Causes can include laryngitis, vocal cord tumour, recurrent laryngeal nerve palsy (e.g. from an apical lung cancer) or gastro-oesophageal reflux.

The face

1. A constricted pupil and a partial ptosis (partial closure of one eyelid) comprise **Horner's syndrome** (p. 232). This can be due to an apical lung tumour compressing the sympathetic nerves in the neck.
2. Look for central **cyanosis** by inspecting the tongue.

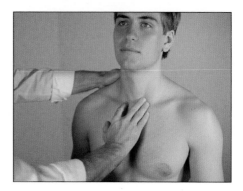

Figure 5.6   Feeling for the position of the trachea.

The trachea

1. Standing in front of the patient, push the forefinger of your right hand very gently up and backwards from the suprasternal notch until the trachea is felt. This examination is uncomfortable for the patient so be gentle. If the trachea is displaced to one side, its edge rather than its middle will be felt and a larger space will be present on one side than the other (see Fig 5.6).
   - Slight displacement to the right is fairly common in healthy people.
   - Significant displacement of the trachea suggests, but is not specific for, disease of the upper lobes of the lung.

2. Feel for a **tracheal tug**—the finger resting on the trachea feels it move inferiorly with each inspiration. This is a sign of gross overexpansion of the chest because of airflow obstruction.

3. Perform the **forced expiratory time test**. Ask the patient to take in a maximum inspiration, then exhale forcefully and completely through the open mouth. You can auscultate over the upper body of the sternum to time exhalation if on a noisy ward.
   - Normal is 3 seconds or less.
   - A forced expiratory time of 9 seconds or more is strongly suggestive of chronic obstructive pulmonary disease in a smoker.

THE CHEST

The chest should be examined anteriorly and posteriorly by **inspection**, **palpation**, **percussion** and **auscultation**. Compare the right and left sides during each part of the examination.

Inspection

1. Look at the shape and symmetry of the chest.
   - When the anteroposterior (AP) diameter is increased compared with the lateral diameter, the chest is described as **barrel-shaped** (see Fig 5.7a). This is an indication of *hyperinflation* of the lungs.
   - **Kyphosis** refers to an exaggerated forward curvature of the spine (see Fig 5.7b).
   - **Scoliosis** is lateral bowing (see Fig 5.7b). Severe thoracic kyphoscoliosis may reduce the lung capacity and increase the work of breathing.
   - Other quite common varieties in chest shape include **pectus excavatum** and **pectus carinatum** (pigeon chest) (see Fig 5.7c and d).
2. Inspect the chest wall for lesions.
   - Look for **scars** from previous thoracic operations, or from chest drains inserted for a previous pneumothorax (often under just below the clavicle) or pleural effusion (usually posterior and basal).
   - **Erythema** and **thickening** of the skin may result from radiotherapy for carcinoma of the lung or lymphoma. Occasionally, radiotherapy can cause burns and skin damage (see Fig 5.8). There is a sharp demarcation between abnormal and normal skin, and small tattoo dots used to delineate the radiation field may be visible.
   - **Subcutaneous emphysema** is a crackling sensation felt on palpating the skin of the chest or neck. It is caused by air tracking from the lungs and is usually due to a pneumothorax.
   - **Prominent veins** may be seen in patients with superior vena caval obstruction.
3. Look at the movement of the chest wall.
   - Look for **asymmetry** of chest wall movement anteriorly and posteriorly.
   - Assessment of expansion of the **upper lobes** is best achieved by inspection from behind the patient, looking

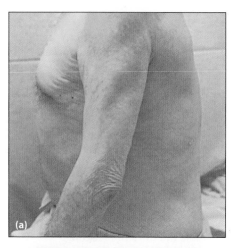

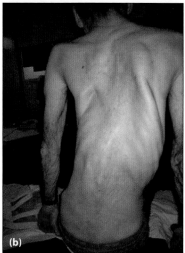

Figure 5.7 Chest shapes. **(a)** Barrel chest: note the increased anteroposterior diameter of the chest. (Epstein O, Perkin D et al. *Clinical Examination*. Elsevier; 2008, Figure 5.36.) **(b)** Very severe kyphosis and scoliosis spinal deformations at an adult age, causing major back pain and contributing to the onset of restrictive respiratory insufficiency. (Laffont I, Tiffreau JM, Yelnik V, Herisson A, Pelissier C. Aging and sequelae of poliomyelitis. *Annals of Physical and Rehabilitation Medicine* 2009; 53(1): 24–33.)

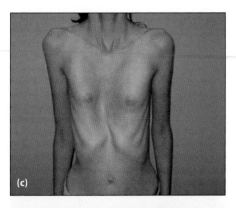

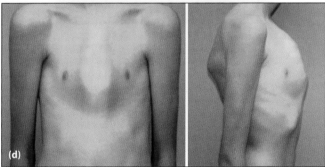

Figure 5.7, continued **(c)** Pectus excavatum in a patient with Marfan's syndrome. (Kotzot D, Schwabegger AH. Etiology of chest wall deformities—a genetic review for the treating physician. *Journal of Pediatric Surgery* 2011; 44(10).) **(d)** Pectus carinatum. (Obermeyer RJ, Goretsky, MJ. Chest wall deformities in pediatric surgery. *Surgical Clinics of North America* 2012; 92(3):669–684.)

down at the clavicles during moderate respiration. The affected side will show delayed or decreased movement.

- For assessment of **lower lobe** expansion, the chest should be assessed from behind by palpation.
- **Reduced chest wall movement on one side** may be due to localised pulmonary fibrosis, consolidation, collapse, pleural effusion or pneumothorax.
- **Bilateral reduction** of chest wall movement indicates a diffuse abnormality, such as chronic obstructive pulmonary disease or diffuse interstitial lung disease.

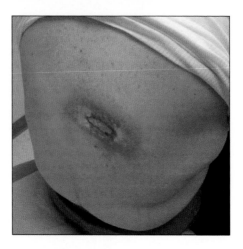

Figure 5.8 Patient who developed Grade 4 skin necrosis from stereotactic body radiation therapy. (Hoppe BS et al. Acute skin toxicity following stereotactic body radiation therapy for stage I non–small-cell lung cancer: Who's at risk? *International Journal of Radiation Oncology Biology Physics* 2008; 72(5), Figure 1.)

Palpation

1. **Chest expansion**.
   - Place your hands firmly on the back of the chest wall with your fingers extending around the sides of the chest. Your thumbs should almost meet in the middle line and should be lifted slightly off the chest so that they are free to move with respiration (see Fig 5.9). As the patient takes a big breath in, your thumbs should move apart symmetrically at least 5 cm. Reduced expansion on one side indicates a lesion of the lobe on that side.
   - Note: Test for Hoover's sign if you suspect COPD. Place your hands around the costal margins of the patient, who is lying in bed. Your thumbs should sit over the xiphisternum, off the skin. Ask the patient to take big breaths in and out. Normally, your thumbs will separate as the patient breathes in. Patients who have COPD have an overexpanded chest and rely on diaphragmatic

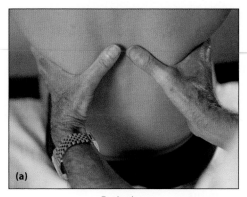

Expiration

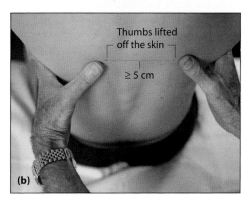

Inspiration

Figure 5.9   Testing chest expansion: normal findings. **(a)** 'Breathe right out.' **(b)** 'Breathe in as far as you can.'

movement to expand the lungs during inspiration. This causes the lower ribs and your thumbs to move inwards: Hoover's sign (see Fig 5.10).

T&O'C examination hint box

The diagnosis of COPD is strongly suggested by a history of cigarette smoking (more than 10 packet years) and a positive Hoover's sign.

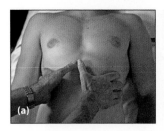 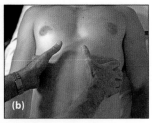

Figure 5.10 Testing for Hoover's sign. **(a)** Expiration. **(b)** Inspiration. Normal findings—Hoover's sign negative.

2. **Vocal fremitus**.
   - Palpate the chest wall with the palm of your hand while the patient says 'ninety-nine' aloud.
   - The front and back of the chest are each palpated in two comparable positions with the palm of one hand on each side of the chest. In this way differences in vibration on the chest wall can be detected.

   This can be a difficult sign to interpret. The causes of change in vocal fremitus are the same as those for vocal resonance (see p. 125).

3. **The ribs**. Gently compress the chest wall anteroposteriorly and laterally. Localised pain suggests a rib fracture, which may be secondary to trauma or may be spontaneous as a result of tumour deposition or primary bone disease.

Percussion

Use the following percussion technique. With your left hand on the chest wall and your fingers slightly separated and aligned with the ribs, press your middle finger firmly against the patient's chest. Use the pad of your right middle finger to firmly strike the middle phalanx of the middle finger of your left hand. Remove the percussing finger quickly so that the note generated is not dampened. The percussing finger must be held partly flexed and a loose swinging movement should come from the wrist and not from the forearm (see Fig 5.11).

1. Percuss the following areas.
   - Percuss on both sides of the anterior, posterior (see Fig 5.12) and axillary regions and in the supraclavicular fossa over the apex of the lung.

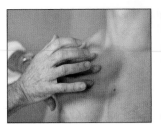 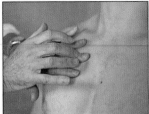

Figure 5.11 Percussion technique.

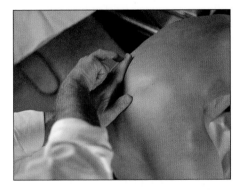

Figure 5.12 Percussing the back.

- Percuss the clavicle directly with the percussing finger.
- For percussion posteriorly, the scapulae can usefully be moved out of the way by asking the patient to move the elbows forwards across the front of the chest.

T&O'C examination hint box

Good percussion technique can only be learnt by practice, and distinguishes the excellent student from the rest. The percussing finger should be flexed at the proximal interphalangeal joint and straight at the distal interphalangeal joint. It should be lifted immediately after it strikes to prevent its deadening the percussion note. Adjust the force of percussion to suit the patient. Do not make a frail elderly woman's percussion note vibrate throughout the hospital.

2. The feel of the percussion note is as important as its sound. The note is affected by the thickness of the chest wall, as well as by underlying structures.
   - Percussion over a solid structure such as the liver or a consolidated area of lung produces a **dull note**.
   - Percussion over a fluid-filled area, such as a pleural effusion, produces an extremely **dull (stony dull) note**.
   - Percussion over the normal lung produces a **resonant note**.
   - Percussion over hollow structures such as the bowel or a pneumothorax produces a **hyper-resonant note**.
3. **Liver dullness**. The upper level of liver dullness is determined by percussing down the anterior chest in the midclavicular line. Normally, this level is over the fifth rib in the right midclavicular line. If the chest is resonant below this level it is a sign of hyperinflation of the lungs, usually due to emphysema or asthma.

Auscultation

Wash your hands and stethoscope (see Fig. 3.1).

1. Using the diaphragm of the stethoscope, listen to the breath sounds in the areas shown in Figure 5.13. It is important to compare one side with the other.
   - Remember to listen high up into the axillae and, using the bell of the stethoscope applied above the clavicles, to listen to the lung apices.
   - Listen for the quality and intensity of the breath sounds and for the presence of additional (adventitious) sounds.
2. *Establish the quality of the breath sounds.* Normal breath sounds are heard with the stethoscope over all parts of the chest. They were once thought to arise in the alveoli (vesicles) of the lungs and are therefore called *vesicular sounds.*
   - **Normal (vesicular) breath sounds** are *louder* and *longer* on *inspiration* than on expiration and there is no gap between the inspiratory and expiratory sounds.
   - **Bronchial breath sounds** are heard when turbulence in the large airways is heard unfiltered by the alveoli. Bronchial breath sounds have a hollow, blowing quality. They are audible throughout expiration and there is often a gap between inspiration and expiration. The

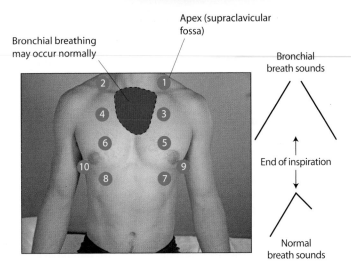

Figure 5.13   Where to auscultate, 1–10.

expiratory sound has a higher intensity and pitch than
the inspiratory sound. They are heard over areas of
consolidation since solid lung conducts the sound of
turbulence in main airways to peripheral areas without
filtering.

3. *Assess the intensity of the breath sounds.* It is better to
   describe breath sounds as being of normal or reduced
   intensity than to speak about air entry. Causes of **reduced**
   breath sounds include:
   • chronic obstructive pulmonary disease
   • pleural effusion (absent breath sounds)
   • pneumothorax (absent breath sounds)
   • a large neoplasm (causing obstruction to a bronchus)
   • pulmonary collapse.

4. *Listen for any added (adventitious) sounds.* There are two
   types of added sounds: continuous (wheezes) and
   interrupted (crackles).
   • **Wheezes** are usually the result of acute or chronic
     obstructive pulmonary disease due to asthma (often
     high-pitched) or chronic obstructive pulmonary disease
     (often low-pitched).

- Interrupted non-musical sounds are best called **crackles**. Note if they are early inspiratory or late or pan-inspiratory:
  - **Early inspiratory crackles of medium coarseness** are suggestive of chronic obstructive pulmonary disease. They differ from those heard in left ventricular failure, which occur later in the respiratory cycle.
  - **Late or pan-inspiratory crackles** suggest disease confined to the alveoli. They may be fine, medium or coarse in quality:
    - ○ **Fine crackles** have been likened to the sound of hair rubbed between the fingers or to the sound Velcro makes when being unstrapped. They are typically caused by interstitial lung disease.
    - ○ **Medium crackles** are often due to left ventricular failure. They can also be present in patients with chronic obstructive pulmonary disease.
    - ○ **Coarse crackles** are characteristic of pools of retained secretions (e.g. bronchiectasis) and have an unpleasant gurgling quality.

5. *Listen for a pleural friction rub.* This occurs when thickened, roughened pleural surfaces rub together as the lungs expand and contract; a continuous or intermittent grating sound may be audible. A pleural rub indicates *pleurisy*, which may be secondary to pulmonary infarction, pneumonia or inflammation of the pleura associated with systemic inflammatory diseases or viral infection.

If a localised abnormality is found on auscultation, try to determine the lobe involved (see Fig 5.1). Further localisation of a mass or opacity on chest x-ray to a bronchopulmonary segment is important and sometimes localised abnormality can be appreciated clinically (see Fig 5.2). Medical students do not need to remember the lung segments for their clinical examination.

T&O'C examination hint box

Medium coarse early inspiratory crackles suggest COPD (usually severe) but should not be used on their own to distinguish left heart failure from COPD.

VOCAL RESONANCE

Auscultation over the chest while the patient speaks gives further information about the lungs' ability to transmit sounds. Ask the patient to say 'ninety-nine' while you listen over each part of the chest.

- Over normal lung the low-pitched components of speech are heard with a booming quality and high-pitched components are attenuated.
- Over consolidated lung the numbers will become clearly audible, whereas over normal lung the sound is muffled.

If vocal resonance is present, bronchial breathing is likely to be heard.

It is important to piece the puzzle together as you examine: it is the combination of disease signs that will guide your provisional diagnosis and next steps (see Table 5.1).

THE HEART

1. Lay the patient at 45° and examine the jugular venous pressure (JVP) for evidence of right heart failure.
2. Palpate and auscultate the praecordium with close attention to the pulmonary component of the second heart sound (P2). This may be palpable or audible with increased intensity at the second intercostal space on the left. It should not be louder than the aortic component, best heard at the right second intercostal space. If P2 is palpable and louder, pulmonary hypertension should be suspected.
3. Feel to the left of the sternum with the heel of your hand for a parasternal impulse (see Fig 5.14)—a sign of right ventricular enlargement.

THE ABDOMEN

Feel for the edge of the liver. It may be palpable below the right costal margin when the lungs are overexpanded or pulsatile if there is tricuspid regurgitation secondary to chronic lung disease.

TABLE 5.1 Comparison of the chest signs in common respiratory diseases

Disorder	Mediastinal displacement	Chest wall movement	Percussion note	Breath sounds	Added sounds
Consolidation	None	Reduced over affected area	Dull	Bronchial	Crackles
Collapse	Ipsilateral shift	Decreased over affected area	Dull	Absent or reduced	Absent
Pleural effusion	Heart displaced to opposite side (trachea displaced only if massive)	Reduced over affected area	Stony dull	Absent over fluid; may be bronchial at upper border	Absent; pleural rub may be found above effusion
Pneumothorax	Tracheal deviation to opposite side if under tension	Decreased over affected area	Resonant	Absent or greatly reduced	Absent
Bronchial asthma	None	Decreased symmetrically	Normal or decreased if severe	Normal or reduced	Wheeze
Interstitial pulmonary fibrosis	None	Decreased symmetrically (minimal)	Normal unaffected by cough or posture	Normal	Fine, late or pan-inspiratory crackles over affected lobes

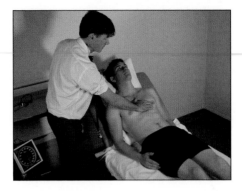

Figure 5.14   Feeling for P2 and parasternal impulse.

T&O'C examination essentials: Dyspnoea

Important differential diagnoses
Respiratory
- Chronic obstructive pulmonary disease (COPD)[1]
- Asthma
- Interstitial lung disease
- Infection (e.g. pneumonia, bronchiectasis)
- Tracheal obstruction
- Pulmonary embolism
- Pneumothorax
- Pleural effusion

Cardiac
- Cardiac failure
- Angina
- Aortic stenosis
- Hypertrophic cardiomyopathy (HCM)
- Mitral stenosis
- Pericardial tamponade

Other
- Obesity
- Loss of physical fitness
- Anaemia
- Anxiety
- Musculoskeletal disease
- Ketoacidosis

---

1 Includes emphysema and chronic bronchitis, and chronic asthma where airflow obstruction is *not* totally reversible.

T&O'C examination hint box 5.1 How to examine the patient complaining of breathlessness

(Wash your hands)
 ! denotes a possible urgent or dangerous problem
1. Make a general inspection for:
   ! • dyspnoea at rest
   ! • use of accessory muscles
   ! • cyanosis
     • sighing respiration (anxiety)
   ! • rapid deep respiration (ketoacidosis)
   ! • lack of respiratory effort, drowsiness (CO_2 narcosis)
     • audible wheeze
     • overexpanded chest
     • obesity
     • anaemia
2. Examine the respiratory system, looking especially for:
   • cough (look at the sputum)
   • clubbing (suppurative lung disease or interstitial lung disease)
   • Hoover's sign
   • fever
   • wheeze
   • bronchial breathing (consolidation)
   • absent breath sounds (pneumothorax, severe asthma)
   • stridor (tracheal obstruction)
3. Examine the cardiovascular system, looking in addition for:
   • hypotension
   • signs of cardiac failure (S3, displaced apex beat, basal crackles, elevated JVP, positive hepatojugular reflux test)
   • aortic stenosis
   • mitral stenosis
   • Kussmaul's sign (pericardial tamponade—associated with severe dyspnoea, hypotension and tachycardia)

The chest OSCE: hints panel

1. This woman has a problem with cough. Take a history from her.
   (a) Ask her about the cough: how long and whether it is productive or not, is getting better or worse, is worse lying down and prevents sleep.
   (b) Ask about the sputum: volume, colour, presence of blood etc.
   (c) Ask about dyspnoea, wheeze and pleuritic chest pain.
   (d) Ask her about any history of known lung disease, including the details.
   (e) Ask her about any current medications.
   (f) Synthesise and present your findings.

2. This man has been breathless. Take an occupational history from him.
   (a) Ask him the following:
       (i) What is your job?
       (ii) What does this involve, in detail? How long have you been doing this work?
       (iii) What ventilation arrangements are provided at work?
       (iv) Are you or other workers or customers permitted to smoke at work?
       (v) Does your work involve exposure to dusts, solvents or animals? (If this is not already clear.)
       (vi) What previous work have you done? What did that involve?
       (vii) Have you any hobbies or pets?
   (b) Present your findings and outline the possible risk associated with any exposure.
3. This man has breathlessness and chest pain made worse by inspiration. Please examine him.
   (Wash your hands and for extra marks your stethoscope)
   (a) If necessary, ask the patient to undress to the waist. Look for wasting and pallor, nail clubbing and cigarette staining of the fingers, and pain on inspiration (pleuritic chest pain).
   (b) Record his respiratory rate and take his temperature.
   (c) Sit him over the side of the bed or ask him to sit upright.
   (d) Stand back and look for central cyanosis (tongue), bruising (trauma) and red raised skin lesions (vasculitis).
   (e) Feel the trachea position. Is it mid-line?
   (f) Examine the chest first from the front and then from the back: inspect, palpate, percuss and auscultate. Note any signs of a friction rub, pneumonia or a pleural effusion.
   (g) Lay the patient at 45° and assess his pulse, blood pressure, JVP and praecordium. (Pulmonary embolus)
   (h) Assess his lower legs for pitting oedema (bilateral) and signs of deep venous thrombosis (unilateral).
   (i) Synthesise and present your findings.
4. This man has haemoptysis and weight loss. Please examine him.
   (Wash your hands)
   (a) Look for obvious evidence of weight loss or cachexia.
   (b) Carefully inspect the nails of his hands for clubbing and look for wrist swelling. (Hypertrophic osteoarthropathy)
   (c) Look for wasting of the small muscles of the hands. (Pancoast tumour)
   (d) Feel for cervical and other lymph node groups.
   (e) Examine his chest systematically.
   (f) Palpate for tracheal deviation.
   (g) Particularly look for unilateral signs that might indicate a lung cancer (e.g. evidence of mediastinal shift, local area of dullness, signs of an effusion).
   (h) Synthesise and present your findings.

T&O'C examination essentials

The chest history and examination

1. Dyspnoea of respiratory cause can sometimes be difficult to distinguish from cardiac dyspnoea, but a careful history can be diagnostic.

2. The smoking history and occupational history are particularly important in any patient with respiratory symptoms.

3. Production of sputum and particularly the presence of haemoptysis must be documented. Available sputum should be inspected.

4. Inspect for chest wall symmetry, palpate for expansion, percuss for dullness and auscultate for abnormal or reduced breath sounds. Examination of the upper lobes should not be forgotten.

5. Although a systematic and complete examination is essential, you may elect to examine the posterior chest (lower lobes) first, since in most cases 'this is where the money is' in respiratory disease.

6. Chronic obstructive pulmonary disease is suggested by a history of smoking, the presence of persistent wheeze, early inspiratory crackles and diminished breath sounds. Test for Hoover's sign and forced expiratory time.

7. An absence of clinical signs does not exclude a respiratory disease; the clinical signs can be less sensitive than investigations such as a chest X-ray (e.g. for detection of a mass lesion) or spirometry (e.g. airflow limitation).

The abdomen

Jaundice is a disease that your friends diagnose.[1]

Sir William Osler (1849–1919)

This chapter presents an introduction to history taking and examination of conditions whose signs are found chiefly in the abdomen. Gastrointestinal, haematological and renal disease can present with abdominal symptoms and signs, and these along with their peripheral signs are all discussed in this chapter.

The gastrointestinal history

When the history suggests a probable gastrointestinal problem, the examination is directed at the gastrointestinal system and begins with the peripheral signs of gut disease, as set out below.

PRESENTING SYMPTOMS (see Box 6.1)

Abdominal pain

Careful history taking will often lead to the correct diagnosis of the cause of abdominal pain. As usual, the following aspects should be considered (SOCRATES):

- **Site.** Ask the patient to point to the site of pain and to where the pain is maximal. Note the areas of the abdomen

---

1 Painless jaundice is classically caused by a pancreatic cancer obstructing the bile duct. The first evidence may be yellow sclera (jaundice) noticed by others, not the patient.

The gastrointestinal system assessment sequence

1. Presenting symptoms (e.g. abdominal pain, loss of weight or appetite, difficulty swallowing, nausea, vomiting, diarrhoea, constipation, rectal bleeding, jaundice)
2. Detailed questions about the presenting symptoms (SOCRATES)
3. Questions about previous gastrointestinal problems, procedures or operations and risk factors (e.g. viral hepatitis, excess alcohol consumption)
4. Examination for peripheral signs of gastrointestinal disease
5. Examination of the abdomen: areas of tenderness, liver and spleen, other masses, ascites, bowel sounds, etc
6. Rectal examination
7. Provisional and differential diagnosis

Box 6.1
The gastrointestinal history: presenting symptoms

Major symptoms
Abdominal pain
Appetite and/or weight change
Nausea and/or vomiting
Heartburn and/or acid regurgitation
Dysphagia
Disturbed defecation (diarrhoea, constipation, faecal incontinence)
Bleeding (haematemesis, melaena, rectal bleeding)
Jaundice
Dark urine, pale stools
Abdominal swelling
Pruritus
Lethargy
Fever

involved (each with a specific name you need to remember; see Fig 6.8 later in the chapter).

- **Onset.** Find out when the pain began and whether the onset was sudden or gradual. Abdominal pain may be an acute (<1 month), subacute (1–6 months) or chronic (>6 months) problem.
- **Character.** Find out what the pain is like (subjective quality e.g. pressure, burning, knife-like etc) and whether it comes and goes or is constant.

- Colicky pain comes and goes in waves and is related to peristaltic movements; it suggests bowel or ureteric obstruction.
- Constant pain may have many causes; for example, pain from biliary tract disease is usually constant and severe—this occurs with a gallstone passing through the bile duct.
- **Radiation.** Ask the patient whether the pain travels elsewhere and, if so, to point to it. For example, pain due to pancreatic disease or a penetrating peptic ulcer (now rare) often radiates through to the back. Pain may radiate to the shoulder with diaphragmatic irritation or to the neck with oesophageal reflux.
- **Alleviating factors.** Ask about factors that seem to make the pain better such as eating, passing stool or taking antacids. Pain due to peptic ulceration may be relieved by meals or taking an antacid (as acid is buffered). Antacids may relieve heartburn from gastro-oesophageal reflux. Defecation or passage of flatus may temporarily relieve the pain of any colonic disease. Patients who obtain some relief by rolling around vigorously are more likely to have a colicky pain from localised bowel disease, whereas those who lie perfectly still are more likely to have peritonitis.
- **Timing.** Find out when the pain began. Determine whether the pain is intermittent or continuous and, if intermittent, whether there is a daily or weekly pattern to the pain:
  - How often do the pain attacks occur?
  - Are they predictable?
  - How long do they last?
- **Exacerbating factors.** Find out whether any factors (eating, passing stool, moving) make the pain worse. For example, eating may precipitate ischaemic pain in the small bowel if the vessels are narrowed (mesenteric angina) and lead to a fear of eating and thus weight loss.
- **Severity.** Ask the patient how much the pain interferes with normal activities and to grade the pain severity from 0 to 10 or using a four-point grading (mild, moderate, severe, very severe).

Patterns of pain

Peptic ulcer disease

- This is classically a dull or burning pain in the epigastrium (see Fig 6.8 later in the chapter) that is relieved by food or antacids and may occur postprandially.
- It is typically episodic and may occur at night, waking the patient from sleep.
- It is not possible to distinguish duodenal ulceration from gastric ulceration clinically.

T&O'C examination hint box

The most common cause of epigastric pain is functional (non-ulcer) dyspepsia, not peptic ulceration. Gastritis refers to stomach inflammation but is **not** a symptom.

Pancreatic pain

- This is often a steady, epigastric pain or ache that may be partly relieved by sitting up and leaning forwards.
- There is often radiation of the pain to the back.

Biliary pain

- Although often called 'biliary colic' in older textbooks, this is rarely colicky. It is usually a severe, constant, epigastric or right upper quadrant pain that can last for hours and occurs episodically and irregularly.
- Cystic duct obstruction from a gallstone often causes epigastric pain. If inflammation of the gallbladder (cholecystitis) then develops, the pain typically shifts to the right upper quadrant and becomes more severe.
- The pain may also radiate across the upper abdomen and around to the right side of the back in the scapular region.

T&O'C examination hint box

Biliary colic is severe, unpredictable, constant pain that typically lasts for hours in the upper abdomen (epigastrium, right hypochondrium); it is not usually colicky pain.

Renal colic
- This is very severe colicky pain superimposed on a background of constant pain in the renal angle, often radiating towards the groin.

Bowel obstruction
- Peri-umbilical colicky pain suggests a small bowel origin but colonic pain can occur anywhere in the abdomen.
- Small bowel obstruction tends to cause more frequent colicky pain (with a cycle every 2–3 minutes) than large bowel obstruction (every 10–15 minutes).
- Bowel obstruction is often associated with vomiting, constipation (failure to pass flatus or stool) and abdominal distension.

Functional bowel disease (irritable bowel syndrome)
- Pain for which no structural cause can be found is common, especially among younger and middle-aged patients with chronic gastrointestinal symptoms.
- Irritable bowel syndrome (IBS) comprises pain, disturbed bowel habit (constipation, diarrhoea or mixed symptoms) and often bloating.
- The abdominal pain is typically relieved by defecation. The onset of pain is associated with a change in stools (e.g. harder or looser, or less or more frequent).
- Its course can be very prolonged but tends to be intermittent, and it may wax and wane over many years.

Appetite or weight change
- The presence of both anorexia (loss of appetite) and weight loss should make one suspicious of an underlying malignancy, but these symptoms may also occur with depression.
- The combination of weight loss with an increased appetite suggests malabsorption of nutrients or a hypermetabolic state (e.g. thyrotoxicosis).

Nausea and vomiting
- Nausea is the sensation of wanting to vomit. There are many gastrointestinal causes (e.g. peptic ulceration or gastric cancer causing pyloric outlet obstruction) and non-gastrointestinal causes (e.g. labyrinthitis, many drugs, migraine, brainstem tumour, renal failure).

- The volume and nature of the vomitus may suggest the gut cause of the problem:
  - Vomiting of large volumes, but infrequently, suggests gastric outlet obstruction.
  - Frequent vomiting of bile or faecal material suggests bowel obstruction.
- The serious student should overcome all feelings of squeamishness and ask patients detailed questions about their vomitus (and, if necessary, faeces). Patients should, however, be discouraged from providing photographs in most cases.[2]

Heartburn and acid regurgitation

- **Heartburn** refers to the presence of a burning pain or discomfort in the retrosternal area due to reflux of acid from the stomach into the oesophagus. Typically, this sensation travels up towards the throat and occurs after meals or is aggravated by bending, stooping or lying supine. Antacids usually relieve the pain, at least transiently.
- **Acid regurgitation** is an acid (sour) taste in the mouth that is due to reflux.
- **Waterbrash** refers to tasteless liquid (saliva) filling the mouth; this can occur in patients with peptic ulceration, but is not usually a symptom of oesophageal reflux.
- Extra-oesophageal manifestations of gastro-oesophageal reflux disease (GORD) can include chest pain, chronic cough, symptoms of asthma, and hoarseness.

Dysphagia

- **Dysphagia** is difficulty swallowing. Such difficulty may occur with solids or liquids.
- If a patient complains of difficulty swallowing, it is important to differentiate painful swallowing from actual difficulty.

---

2 The Bristol Stool Chart is a visual tool for grading stool from type 1 (separate hard lumps like nuts) to type 7 (watery, no solid bits). Trust the British! The scale objectively correlates with intestinal transit, so looking at stools is useful for assessing gut function too.

- Painful swallowing is termed **odynophagia** and occurs with any severe inflammatory process involving the oesophagus.
- If the patient complains of difficulty initiating swallowing or complains of fluid regurgitating into the nose or choking on trying to swallow, this suggests that the cause of the dysphagia is in the pharynx (**pharyngeal dysphagia**).
- If the patient complains of food sticking after swallowing, it is important to consider causes of oesophageal blockage (e.g. carcinoma or stricture). If the patient also has frequent heartburn, this suggests a stricture caused by oesophagitis.
- If there has been significant weight loss with progressive (worsening) dysphagia, this suggests cancer.
- A history of **intermittent food impaction** suggests the allergic disease eosinophilic oesophagitis.

> ### T&O'C examination hint box
>
> Difficulty swallowing that is described as food sticking and that is progressive and worse with solids is a red flag symptom. Carcinoma of the oesophagus must be considered in these patients.

Diarrhoea

- Diarrhoea can be defined in a number of ways. Patients may complain of frequent stools (more than three per day being abnormal) or they may complain of a change in the consistency of the stools, which have become loose (soft, fluffy) or watery.
- When a history of diarrhoea is obtained, it is important to determine whether this has occurred acutely (<1 month) or is a chronic problem.
- Acute diarrhoea is more likely to be infectious in nature, while chronic diarrhoea has a large number of causes. Consider, in chronic cases:
  - *Secretory diarrhoea.* The stools are of large volume (often more than 1 L a day) and the diarrhoea persists when the patient is fasting. Secretory diarrhoea may be caused by a villous adenoma or, rarely, a tumour that secretes vasoactive intestinal peptide (VIP).

- *Osmotic diarrhoea.* The diarrhoea disappears when the patient fasts (e.g. due to lactose intolerance or the taking of a non-absorbed osmotic laxative).
- *Exudative diarrhoea.* The stools are of small volume but frequent and there is associated blood or mucus (e.g. colon cancer or inflammatory bowel disease).
- *Malabsorption.* If there is steatorrhoea (excess fat in the stools), the stools are pale, foul-smelling and difficult to flush away (e.g. from chronic pancreatitis, coeliac sprue).
- *Increased intestinal motility* (e.g. thyrotoxicosis). Here the stools may be normal in consistency and an increased bowel frequency may not be volunteered as a symptom.

Constipation

- It is important to determine what patients mean if they say they are constipated. Constipation is a common symptom and can refer to the passage of infrequent stools (fewer than three times per week is abnormal), or hard stools or lumpy stools that are difficult to evacuate (i.e. require excessive straining).
- This symptom may occur acutely or it may be a chronic problem. Chronic causes include:
  - colonic obstruction (e.g. cancer)
  - metabolic disease (e.g. hypothyroidism, diabetes mellitus)
  - rectal outlet blockage (e.g. from a failure to relax the external anal sphincter on straining).

Mucus

- The passage of mucus (white flecks on the stool) may occur in inflammatory bowel disease or irritable bowel syndrome, or with rectal carcinomas or villous adenomas.

Bleeding

- Patients may present with:
  - haematemesis (vomiting blood)
  - melaena (passage of jet-black stools from altered blood in the colon)
  - haematochezia (passage of bright-red blood per rectum).

- Bright-red blood on the outside of the stool suggests outlet bleeding (e.g. from haemorrhoids), whereas blood mixed in the stool suggests colonic disease.
- With occult bleeding from the bowel, patients may just present with symptoms and signs of anaemia (e.g. fatigue and pallor) from iron deficiency.

Jaundice

- Usually the patient's relatives notice a yellow discolouration of the sclera or skin due to bilirubin deposition before the patient does.

T&O'C examination hint box

A careful history and examination will reveal the correct diagnosis of the cause of jaundice in two-thirds of patients.

- Ask about other symptoms, including:
  - abdominal pain—gallstones, for example, can cause biliary pain and jaundice
  - changes in the colour of the stools and urine— obstructive jaundice (e.g. blockage of the common bile duct by a gallstone or carcinoma of the pancreas) causes dark urine and pale stools, whereas haemolytic anaemia is associated with dark urine and normal-coloured stools (learn the bilirubin pathway to understand why)
  - fever and malaise (e.g. viral hepatitis or drug reactions).

DRUG AND TREATMENT HISTORY, AND PAST HISTORY

Ask about:
- surgical procedures and current medications
- blood transfusions and anaesthetics
- any diagnosis of previous abdominal disease, including inflammatory bowel disease, and any treatment received
- use of non-steroidal anti-inflammatory drugs (NSAIDs) that can cause ulcers and bleeding.

SOCIAL HISTORY

Ask about:

- the patient's occupation (e.g. healthcare worker exposed to hepatitis)
- recent travel (e.g. to countries where hepatitis is endemic)
- alcohol intake (causes liver, pancreatic and gut disease)
- contact with people who have been jaundiced
- use of intravenous drugs (risk of hepatitis B or C).

FAMILY HISTORY

A family history of colon or gastric cancer, inflammatory bowel disease or liver disease is often relevant.

Examination anatomy

A knowledge of the underlying structures of the abdomen helps explain the various examination techniques. As with the chest examination, try to picture the structures that lie beneath the surface of the area being examined (see Fig 6.1).

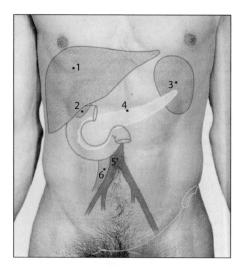

Figure 6.1 The abdominal organs. 1 = liver; 2 = gall bladder; 3 = spleen; 4 = pancreas; 5 = aortic bifurcation; 6 = inferior vena cava.

Examining the gastrointestinal system

See Box 6.2.

Box 6.2
The gastrointestinal system examination sequence

1. General inspection
2. Hands
3. Arms
4. Face
5. Abdomen
6. Chest
7. Back
8. Legs

GENERAL INSPECTION

Look for wasting (malabsorption, anorexia or malignancy), obesity, jaundice or rashes.

1. Fragile vesicles appear on exposed areas of the skin and heal with scarring in patients with porphyria cutanea tarda, a genetic disease that causes cirrhosis and is more common in those with hepatitis C.
2. Tense tethering of the skin in systemic sclerosis may be associated with heartburn and dysphagia from gastro-oesophageal reflux and diarrhoea from gastrointestinal motility disorders.

THE HANDS AND NAILS

Pick up the patient's right hand, then the left.

1. Look for any rash.
2. Note any changes of **arthritis**. Arthropathy of the second and third metacarpophalangeal joints may be present in the hands of patients with the iron-storage disease **haemochromatosis**.
3. Look for leuconychia and clubbing. When chronic liver or kidney disease results in hypoalbuminaemia, the nail beds opacify, often leaving only a rim of pink nail bed at the top of the nail (leuconychia [white nails]). Up to one-third of patients with cirrhosis may have finger clubbing.

4. Look for **purpura**, which is really any sort of bruising. The lesions can vary in size from pinheads called **petechiae** to large bruises called **ecchymoses**, as occurs in liver disease. If the petechiae are raised (**palpable purpura**), this suggests an underlying systemic vasculitis or bacteraemia.

Palms

1. **Palmar erythema ('liver palms')** is reddening of the palms of the hands affecting the thenar and hypothenar eminences. Often the soles of the feet are also affected. This can be a feature of chronic liver disease.
2. Inspect the palmar creases for pallor suggesting anaemia, which may result from gastrointestinal blood loss, malabsorption (folate, vitamin B_{12}), haemolysis (e.g. hypersplenism) or chronic systemic disease.
3. **Dupuytren's contracture** is a visible and palpable thickening and contraction of the palmar fascia causing permanent flexion, most often of the ring finger. It is often bilateral and occasionally may affect the feet. It is associated with alcoholism (not liver disease), but is also found in some manual workers and may be familial.

Hepatic flap (asterixis)

Ask the patient to stretch out the arms in front, separate the fingers and extend the wrists for 15 seconds. Jerky, irregular flexion–extension movement at the wrist and metacarpophalangeal joints, often accompanied by lateral movements of the fingers, constitutes the flapping of hepatic encephalopathy in liver failure.

ARMS

1. At the **wrist** and **forearms**, inspect for **scars**.
2. Inspect the upper limbs for **bruising**. Large bruises (ecchymoses) may be due to clotting abnormalities (e.g. in chronic liver disease).
3. Look for **muscle wasting**, which is often a late manifestation of malnutrition in alcoholic patients. Alcohol can also cause a proximal myopathy.
4. **Scratch marks** due to severe itch (pruritus) are often prominent in patients with obstructive or cholestatic jaundice.

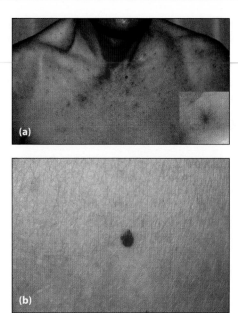

Figure 6.2   **(a)** Spider telangiectasias (naevi) on the upper aspect of the chest associated with alcohol abuse. The inset shows a spider telangiectasia with a central erythematous macule and surrounded by radiating vessels. (Liu SW, Lien MH, Fenske, NA. The effects of alcohol and drug abuse on the skin. *Clinics in Dermatology* 2010; 28(1), Figure 1.) **(b)** Cherry haemangioma—a discreet, smooth-surfaced, deep-red papule on the trunk. (Brinster NK, Liu V, Diwan AH, McKee PH. *Dermatopathology: High-Yield Pathology*. Elsevier; 2011, Figure 1.)

5. **Spider naevi** consist of a central arteriole from which radiate numerous small vessels that look like spiders' legs (see Fig 6.2a). They range in size from just visible to 0.5 cm in diameter. Their usual distribution is in the area drained by the superior vena cava, so they are found on the arms, neck and chest wall. Pressure applied with a pointed object to the central arteriole causes blanching of the whole lesion. Rapid refilling occurs on release of the pressure. The finding of more than two spider naevi anywhere on the body is likely to be abnormal except during pregnancy. Spider naevi can be caused by cirrhosis, most frequently

due to alcohol. They can easily be distinguished from **Campbell de Morgan spots (cherry angiomas)**, which are flat or slightly elevated red circular spots that occur on the abdomen or the front of the chest (see fig 6.2b). They do not blanch on pressure and are very common and harmless.

THE FACE

Eyes

1. Look first at the sclerae for signs of **jaundice** or **anaemia**.
2. A red eye from **iritis** (p. 230) may be seen in inflammatory bowel disease.
3. Conjunctival pallor suggests anaemia and is more reliable than examination of the nail beds or palmar creases.

Salivary glands

1. The normal **parotid gland** is impalpable; enlargement leads to a swelling in the cheek behind the angle of the jaw and in the upper neck (see Fig 6.3). Examine for signs of inflammation (warmth, tenderness, redness and swelling) and decide whether the facial swelling is lumpy or not (see Fig 6.4).
   - Alcoholic liver disease can cause bilateral parotid swelling.

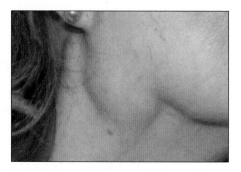

Figure 6.3   Parotid enlargement. (Rich R et al. *Clinical Immunology*. Elsevier; 2013, Fig. 53.3.)

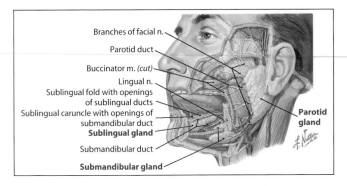

Branches of facial n.
Parotid duct
Buccinator m. (cut)
Lingual n.
Sublingual fold with openings
of sublingual ducts
Sublingual caruncle with openings of
submandibular duct
Sublingual gland
Submandibular duct
Submandibular gland
Parotid gland

Figure 6.4   Anatomy of the salivary glands.

- A mixed parotid tumour (a pleomorphic adenoma) is the most common cause of a lump. Parotid carcinoma may cause a facial nerve palsy (p. 198).
2. Feel in the mouth (wear a glove!) for a parotid calculus, which may be present at the parotid duct orifice (opposite the upper second molar). Mumps also causes acute parotid enlargement, which is usually bilateral.
3. **Submandibular gland** enlargement is most often due to a calculus. This may be palpable bimanually. Place your index finger on the floor of the mouth beside the tongue, feeling between it and fingers placed behind the body of the mandible. It may also be enlarged in chronic liver disease.

Mouth

1. Look first briefly at the state of the teeth and note whether they are real or false. False teeth will have to be removed for complete examination of the mouth. Loose-fitting false teeth may be responsible for ulcers, and decayed teeth may be responsible for fetor.
2. **Fetor hepaticus** is a sweet smell of the breath and is an indication of hepatocellular failure.
3. Thickened epithelium with bacterial debris and food particles commonly cause a **coating** over the tongue, especially in smokers. It is rarely a sign of disease.

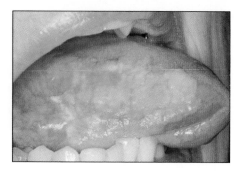

Figure 6.5 Large leukoplakia on the lateral border of the tongue. (Huber MA. White oral lesions, actinic cheilitis, and leukoplakia: confusions in terminology and definition: Facts and controversies. *Clinics in Dermatology* 2010; 28(3), Figure 8.)

4. **Leucoplakia** is white-coloured thickening of the mucosa of the tongue and mouth (see Fig 6.5); the condition is premalignant. Most of the causes of leucoplakia begin with 'S'—sore teeth (poor dental hygiene), smoking, spirits, sepsis or syphilis—but often no cause is apparent.

5. The term **glossitis** is generally used to describe a smooth appearance of the tongue, which may also be erythematous. The appearance is due to atrophy of the papillae, and in later stages there may be shallow ulceration. These changes occur in the tongue often as a result of nutritional deficiencies (e.g. vitamin B_{12}, folate or iron).

6. **Aphthous ulceration** is common. It begins as a small painful vesicle on the tongue or mucosal surface of the mouth, which may break down to form a painful shallow ulcer with surrounding erythema. These ulcers heal without scarring. They usually do not indicate any serious underlying systemic disease, but may occur in Crohn's disease or coeliac disease.

7. Fungal infection with *Candida albicans* (thrush) causes creamy white, curd-like patches in the mouth or on the tongue, which are removed only with difficulty and leave a bleeding surface. These can be associated with immune deficiency (e.g. human immunodeficiency virus [HIV] infection).

8. Look for:
   - hypertrophy of the gums, which may occur with infiltration by leukaemic cells, especially in cases of acute monocytic leukaemia
   - gum bleeding, ulceration, infection
   - haemorrhage of the buccal and pharyngeal mucosa
   - telangiectasias on the lips and tongue (which may be a sign of hereditary haemorrhagic telangiectasia that may be a cause of occult bleeding in the bowel).

THE ABDOMEN

The abdomen should be examined by inspection, palpation, percussion and auscultation. The abdominal examination includes an examination of the groin and the rectum if clinically indicated.

Inspection

The patient should **lie flat**, but make sure this is not uncomfortable for the patient and in an exam ask if it is alright for you to lay the patient flat (see Fig 6.6). Place one pillow under the patient's head and ensure the abdomen is exposed from the nipples to the pubic symphysis.

1. Begin with a careful look for abdominal **scars**, which may indicate previous surgery or trauma. Look in the area around the umbilicus for small laparoscopic surgical scars. Older scars are white, whereas recent scars are pink because the tissue remains vascular.

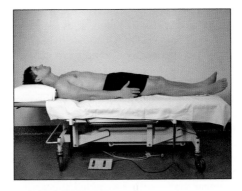

Figure 6.6 Abdominal examination: positioning the patient.

2. Note the presence of **stomas** (colostomy, ileostomy or ileal conduit), fistulae or a peritoneal dialysis catheter.
3. Generalised abdominal **distension** may be present. All the causes of this sound as though they begin with the letter 'F':
   - fat (gross obesity)
   - fluid (ascites)
   - fetus
   - flatus (gaseous distension due to bowel obstruction)
   - faeces
   - filthy big tumour (e.g. large polycystic kidneys or an ovarian tumour)
   - phantom pregnancy (looks pregnant but isn't).

   When the peritoneal cavity is filled with large volumes of fluid (ascites) from whatever cause, the abdominal flanks and wall appear tense and the umbilicus is shallow or everted and points downwards.
4. **Local swellings** may indicate enlargement of one of the abdominal or pelvic organs or weakening of the abdominal wall as a result of previous surgery (**incisional hernia**).
5. Prominent **veins** may be obvious on the abdominal wall in patients with severe portal hypertension or inferior vena cava obstruction.
6. **Pulsations** may be visible. An expanding central pulsation in the epigastrium suggests an abdominal aortic aneurysm. However, the abdominal aorta can often be seen to pulsate in thin healthy people.
7. **Visible peristalsis** usually suggests intestinal obstruction.
8. **Skin lesions** should also be noted. These include:
   - vesicles of herpes zoster, which occur in a radicular pattern (they are localised to only one side of the abdomen in the distribution of a single nerve root; herpes zoster may be responsible for severe abdominal pain that is of mysterious origin until the rash appears)
   - skin tattoos, which may indicate an increased risk of hepatitis B or C infection
   - stretching of the abdominal wall severe enough to cause rupture of the elastic fibres in the skin, which produces pink linear marks with a wrinkled appearance called **striae**. When these are wide and purple-coloured,

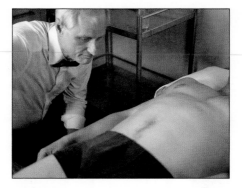

Figure 6.7   Inspecting the abdomen: approved posture.

Cushing's syndrome (from steroid hormone excess) may be the cause. Ascites and pregnancy are much more common causes of striae.

9. Next, squat down beside the bed so that the patient's abdomen is at eye level (see Fig 6.7). Ask the patient to take slow deep breaths through the mouth and watch for the movement of a large liver in the right upper quadrant (see below) or spleen in the left upper quadrant. Ask the patient to cough and look for the reducible swellings that indicate hernias. These may be present under scars (incisional hernias) or in the inguinal region.

Palpation

Reassure the patient that the examination will not be painful and use warm hands. Ask whether any particular area is tender and examine this area last.

For descriptive purposes the abdomen is divided into nine regions, or four quadrants (see Fig 6.8). Palpation in each region is performed with the palmar surface of the fingers acting together. For palpation of the edges of organs or masses, the lateral surface of the forefinger is the most sensitive part of the hand.

1. Begin with **light pressure** in each region. Stop straight away if this causes pain for the patient. All the movements of your hand should occur at the metacarpophalangeal joints and your hand should be moulded to the shape of

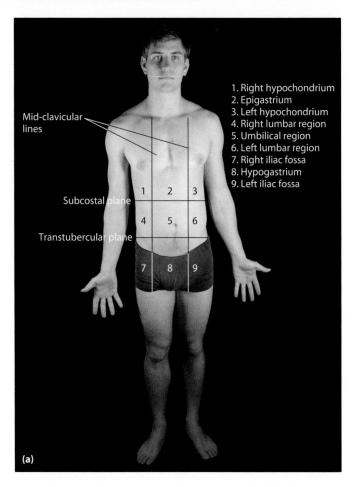

Figure 6.8 **(a)** Regions of the abdomen. The subcostal plane is an imaginary line joining the lowest parts of the rib cage (10th costal cartilage). The transtubercular plane is a line joining the tubercles of the iliac crests.

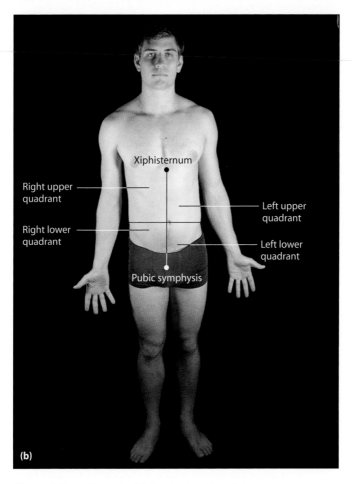

(b)

Figure 6.8, continued   (b) Quadrants of the abdomen.

> **Box 6.3**
> **Descriptive features of intra-abdominal masses**
>
> For any abdominal mass *all* of the following should be determined:
> - site: the region involved and the depth (abdominal wall or intra-abdominal)
> - size (which should be measured) and shape
> - tenderness (yes or no)
> - surface, which may be regular or irregular
> - edge, which may be regular or irregular
> - consistency, which may be hard or soft
> - mobility and movement with inspiration
> - whether it is pulsatile or not
> - whether one can get above the mass.

the abdominal wall. Note the presence of any tenderness or masses in each region.

2. Next perform **deep palpation**. Deep palpation is used to detect deeper masses and to define those already discovered. Ask the patient about tenderness. Any mass must be characterised and described (see Box 6.3).

- **Guarding** of the abdomen, when resistance to palpation occurs due to contraction of the abdominal muscles, may result from tenderness or anxiety, and may be voluntary or **involuntary**. The latter suggests peritonitis.

- **Rigidity** is a constant involuntary contraction of the abdominal muscles always associated with tenderness and indicates peritoneal irritation.

- **Rebound tenderness** is said to be present when the abdominal wall, having been compressed slowly, is released rapidly and a sudden stab of pain results. This may make the patient wince, so watch the patient's face while this manoeuvre is performed. It strongly suggests the presence of peritonitis. If the abdomen is very tender, light percussion will give the same information and cause less discomfort.

- **Referred tenderness** is where palpation in a non-tender area causes pain in another area. An example is Rovsing's sign (press in the left lower quadrant—if pain occurs in the right lower quadrant, this suggests acute appendicitis in a patient with a typical history).

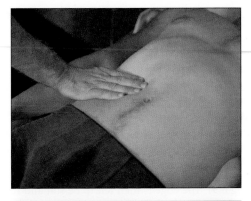

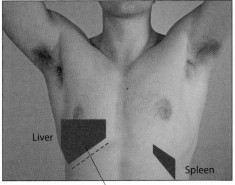

Liver

Spleen

Descent of liver
with inspiration
(↑ dullness)

Figure 6.9   Abdominal examination: the liver.

- **Cough tenderness** (localised pain in the abdomen on coughing) is another sign of peritonitis.

Liver

1. Feel for hepatomegaly (see Fig 6.9). With your examining hand aligned parallel to the right costal margin, and beginning in the right iliac fossa, ask the patient to breathe in and out slowly through the mouth. With each expiration advance your hand closer to the right costal margin by 1 or

2 cm. During inspiration keep your hand still while the lateral margin of the forefinger waits expectantly for the liver edge to strike it.

2. If the liver is palpable, its surface should be felt. The edge of the liver and the surface itself may be:
    - hard or soft
    - tender or non-tender
    - regular or irregular
    - pulsatile or non-pulsatile (it will usually be pulsatile if there is tricuspid regurgitation).

    The normal liver edge may be palpable just below the right costal margin on deep inspiration, especially in thin people (see Fig 6.9). The edge is then felt to be soft and regular with a fairly sharply defined border, and the surface of the liver itself is smooth.

3. If the liver edge is palpable, the total **liver span** should be measured. The normal upper border of the liver is level with the fifth rib in the midclavicular line. At this point the percussion note over the chest changes from resonant to dull (p. 153). To estimate the liver span, percuss down along the right midclavicular line until the liver dullness is encountered and measure from here to the palpable liver edge. The normal span is less than 13 cm.

4. A pulsatile liver comes down to bump the examiner's hand in time with the heartbeat.

Gall bladder

1. The gall bladder is occasionally palpable below the right costal margin where this crosses the lateral border of the rectus muscles, but this does not occur in health.

2. If biliary obstruction or gall bladder disease is suspected, orient your examining hand perpendicular to the costal margin, feeling from medial to lateral. Unlike the liver edge, the gall bladder, if palpable, will be a bulbous, focal rounded mass that moves downwards on inspiration.

3. **Murphy's sign** should be sought if cholecystitis is suspected. While taking a deep breath in, the patient catches his or her breath when an inflamed gall bladder presses on the examiner's hand, which is lying at the costal margin.

Spleen

1. The spleen enlarges inferiorly and medially. Its edge should be sought below the umbilicus in the mid-line initially.

2. A **two-handed technique** is recommended (see Fig 6.10). Place your left hand posterolaterally just below the left lower ribs and your right hand on the abdomen parallel to the left costal margin. Don't start palpation too near the costal margin or a large spleen will be missed. As you advance your right hand closer to the left costal margin, compress your left hand firmly over the rib cage so as to produce a loose fold of skin; this removes tension from the abdominal wall and enables a slightly enlarged soft spleen to be felt as it moves down towards the right iliac fossa at the end of inspiration.

3. If the spleen is not palpable, roll the patient onto the right side towards you and repeat the process, beginning close to the left costal margin.

Kidneys

An attempt to palpate both of the kidneys should be routine even in the gastrointestinal examination—because you may confuse a kidney for the spleen or even the liver!

1. Use a **bimanual method**. Lay the patient flat on his or her back. To palpate the right kidney, slide your hand underneath the patient's back to rest with the heel of your

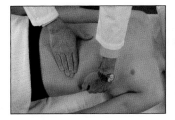
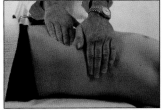

Figure 6.10 Palpation of the spleen. Palpation begins in the lower mid-abdomen and finishes up under the left costal margin. Your hand supports the patient's side ... and then rests over the lower costal margin to reduce skin resistance. If the spleen is not palpable when the patient is flat, the patient should be rolled towards you and two-handed palpation repeated.

hand under the right loin. Your fingers remain free to flex at the metacarpophalangeal joints in the area of the renal angle. The flexing fingers can push the contents of the abdomen anteriorly. Place your other hand over the right upper quadrant and try to palpate the left kidney (see Fig 6.11).

2. When ballotting the kidneys, the renal angle is pressed sharply by the flexing fingers of your posterior hand, which must be positioned under the patient almost to the spine in the middle line. The kidney can be felt to float upwards and strike the anterior hand.

3. The lower pole of the right kidney may be palpable in thin people. Both kidneys move downwards only a little with inspiration.

T&O'C examination hint box

It is common to **confuse** a **large left kidney** with an **enlarged spleen**. Know the way to distinguish them. The major distinguishing features are:

- The spleen has no palpable upper border—you cannot feel the space between the spleen and the costal margin, which is present in renal enlargement.
- The spleen, unlike the kidney, has a notch anteromedially, which may be palpable.
- The spleen moves inferomedially on inspiration, whereas the kidney moves inferiorly.
- The spleen is not usually ballottable unless gross ascites is present, but the kidney is, again because of its retroperitoneal position.
- The percussion note is dull over the spleen but is usually resonant over the kidney, because the latter lies posterior to loops of gas-filled bowel.
- A friction rub may occasionally be heard over the spleen, but never over the kidney, because it is too posterior.

Percussion

Percussion is used to define the size and nature of organs and masses, and to detect fluid in the peritoneal cavity. It is reliable for the detection of an enlarged liver and may be more sensitive than palpation for detecting a mildly enlarged spleen.

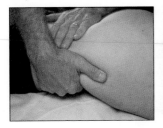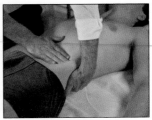

Figure 6.11   Ballotting the left kidney.

1. Percuss over the lowest intercostal space in the left anterior axillary line, in both inspiration and expiration, with the patient supine.
2. Splenomegaly should be suspected if the percussion note is dull or becomes dull on complete inspiration.
3. To test for ascites, begin with percussion starting in the mid-line with the finger pointing towards the feet; the percussion note is tested out towards the flanks on each side.
4. If dullness in the flanks is detected, the sign of **shifting dullness** should be sought (see Fig 6.12). Stand on the right side of the bed and percuss out to the left flank until dullness is reached. Mark this point with a finger or pen (not an indelible one) and ask the patient to roll towards you. After 30 seconds or so repeat percussion over the marked point. If fluid shifts, the dullness will disappear. Shifting dullness is present if the area of dullness has changed to become resonant and indicates ascites.

Auscultation

Listen for bowel sounds, bruits and rubs.

1. Place the diaphragm of the stethoscope just below the umbilicus. In healthy people, bowel sounds can be heard over all parts of the abdomen. They have a soft, gurgling character and occur only intermittently.
   - Bowel sounds should be described as **present** or **absent**.
   - Complete absence of bowel sounds (over a 3-minute period with the stethoscope in one place) indicates **paralytic ileus**.

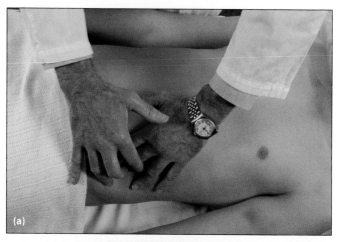

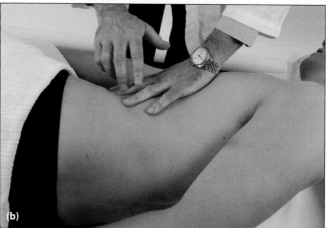

Figure 6.12 Shifting dullness. **(a)** Percuss out to the left flank until the percussion note becomes dull. Mark this spot with your finger. **(b)** Roll the patient towards you, wait 30 seconds. Shifting dullness is present if the left lateral dull area is now resonant.

- An obstructed bowel produces a louder, more high-pitched sound with a **tinkling** quality, which is due to the presence of air and liquid ('obstructed bowel sounds').
- Intestinal hurry or rush, which may occur in diarrhoeal states, causes loud gurgling sounds (borborygmi), which are often audible without the stethoscope. Borborygmi may be loud enough to interfere with the more important auscultation of the heart.

2. **Abdominal bruits** (high-pitched, mostly systolic sounds) may be audible over the liver in the presence of hepatocellular cancer.
   - Continuous sounds may be caused by arteriovenous shunts related to portal hypertension.
   - Renal bruits (heard on either side of the mid-line above the umbilicus) may indicate renal artery stenosis, but soft abdominal bruits are a common normal finding.
3. A **friction rub** (creaking or grating noise) may be audible as the patient breathes in and out when the peritoneum is inflamed. This rare sign may be the result of a hepatic or splenic infarct, or of malignant deposits.

The groin

In all patients with an acute abdomen, a strangulated hernia must be excluded as a cause. If a hernia is not obvious while the patient is lying down, complete examination requires that the patient be examined while standing. A summary of the relevant surface anatomy is shown in Figure 6.13.

Technique

1. Wash your hands, glove up and position the patient.
2. Inspect the patient standing up. Ask the patient to point to the lump and then cough, then palpate over the region.
3. Ask the patient to lie down and re-examine him or her (inspect and palpate).
4. Try to distinguish an inguinal hernia from a femoral hernia (often difficult).
5. In men, examine the testes and scrotum to complete your examination.

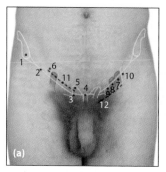

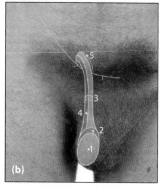

Inguinal region: bones and soft tissues
1 Anterior superior iliac spine
2 Inguinal ligament
3 Pubic tubercle
4 Symphysis pubis
5 Superficial inguinal ring
6 Deep inguinal ring
7 Femoral artery
8 Femoral vein
9 Femoral canal
10 Femoral nerve
11 Inguinal hernia incision
12 Femoral hernia incision

Testis and spermatic cord
1 Testis
2 Superior pole of epididymis
3 Spermatic cord
4 Vas deferens
5 Superficial inguinal ring

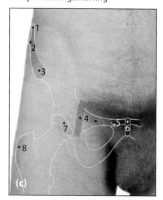

Pelvis and anterior thigh: palpable structures
1 Iliac crest
2 Tubercle of ilium
3 Anterior superior iliac spine
4 Femoral artery
5 Pubic tubercle
6 Symphysis pubis
7 Head of femur
8 Greater trochanter

Figure 6.13 Surface anatomy of the groin and key structures.

Inguinal hernia

1. An **inguinal hernia** typically bulges *above* the crease of the groin. Confirm the position of the swelling in the groin above or below the inguinal ligament, which lies between the anterior superior iliac spine and the pubic tubercle. The pubic tubercle is found just above the attachment of the adductor longus tendon to the pubic bone, which can be felt on the upper medial aspect of the thigh (see Fig 6.13). If the swelling lies *medial to* and *above* the pubic tubercle, it is likely to be an inguinal hernia (see Fig 6.14a).

2. The characteristic inguinal hernia is a soft lump that can usually be pushed back into the abdominal cavity (i.e. it is reducible), and an impulse is palpable if the patient coughs. The cough impulse must always be sought.

    - An **indirect inguinal hernia** passes through the internal inguinal ring, which lies 2 cm above the midpoint of the inguinal ligament, just above and lateral to the femoral pulse, and descends through the inguinal canal. In males a small indirect inguinal hernia may be palpated by gently invaginating the scrotum and feeling an impulse at the external ring when the patient coughs (see Fig 6.14b). When examining a male, remember to count the number of testes in the scrotum (normally two) as a maldescended testis may be confused with an inguinal hernia.

    - A **direct inguinal hernia** protrudes forwards through the inguinal (Hesselbach's) triangle. A direct inguinal hernia usually appears immediately with standing (and coughing or straining) and disappears on lying down.

Femoral hernia

1. A **femoral hernia** usually bulges *into the groin crease* at its *medial* end. Hence, these occur *lateral to* and *below* the pubic tubercle, 2 cm medial to the femoral pulse, and do not involve the inguinal canal.

2. Do not confuse an impulse conducted by the femoral vein (saphena varix) during coughing with a femoral hernia. A femoral hernia is usually small and firm and can be mistaken for a lymph node.

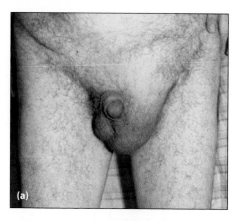

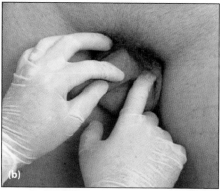

Figure 6.14 **(a)** Note the elliptical swelling of an indirect inguinal hernia descending into the scrotum on the right side. Also note the globular swelling of a direct inguinal hernia on the left side. **(b)** To examine the inguinal canal in a male, invaginate the scrotum as shown (always wear gloves). (Swartz M. *Textbook of Physical Diagnosis*. Elsevier; 2014, Figure 15.31.)

3. If a hernia strangulates (bowel caught in the hernia has its blood supply cut off), the overlying skin may become red and tense, and the lump is usually tender. The cough impulse is lost.

T&O'C examination hint box

Remember that:
- hernias are often bilateral
- two different types may occur on the same side
- there may be an associated **hydrocele** (increased fluid in the tunica vaginalis causing scrotal swelling).

Incisional hernia

1. Any abdominal scar may be the site of a hernia because of abdominal wall weakness. Assess this by asking the patient to cough while you look for abnormal bulges.
2. Next have the patient lift his or her head and shoulders off the bed while your hand rests on the forehead and resists this movement.
3. If a bulge is seen, your other hand should palpate for a fascial layer defect in the muscle.

Rectal examination

Explain to the patient what is to happen and obtain permission.

1. Lie the patient on his or her left side with the knees drawn up and the back facing you. This is called the left lateral position.
2. Don a pair of gloves and begin inspection of the anus and perianal area by separating the buttocks.
3. Note the presence of thrombosed external haemorrhoids (piles: small [<1 cm], tense bluish swellings seen on one side of the anal margin) or skin tags (these look like tags elsewhere on the body and can be an incidental finding or occur with haemorrhoids or Crohn's disease).
4. Lubricate the tip of your gloved right index finger and place it over the anus. Ask the patient to breathe in and out quietly through the mouth, as a distraction and to aid relaxation. Slowly apply increasing pressure with the pulp of your finger until you feel the sphincter relax slightly. Then advance your finger slowly into the rectum. At this

stage sphincter tone should be assessed as increased, normal or reduced.

5. First perform palpation of the anterior wall of the rectum for the **prostate gland** in the male and for the cervix in the female. The normal prostate is a firm, rubbery bilobed mass with a central furrow. The presence of a very hard nodule suggests carcinoma of the prostate. The prostate is boggy and tender in patients with prostatitis.

6. Then rotate your finger clockwise so that the left lateral wall, posterior wall and right lateral wall of the rectum can be palpated in turn. Advance your finger as high as possible into the rectum and slowly withdraw it along the rectal wall.

7. After you withdraw your finger, inspect the glove for bright blood or melaena, mucus or pus, and note the colour of the faeces.

T&O'C examination hint box

- Haemorrhoids are not palpable unless thrombosed.
- The occurrence of significant pain during rectal examination suggests an anal fissure, an ischiorectal abscess, a recently thrombosed external haemorrhoid, proctitis or anal ulceration.

THE CHEST

In males, **gynaecomastia** or enlargement of the breasts may be a sign of chronic liver disease. Tender gynaecomastia is common when patients take the drug spironolactone.

THE BACK

1. Strike the vertebral column gently with the base of the fist to elicit bony tenderness. This may be due to malignant deposits.

2. Look for sacral oedema in a patient confined to bed (e.g. from nephrotic syndrome or congestive cardiac failure).

THE LEGS

1. Note oedema, which can occur with ascites (low albumin).

2. **Pruritus** (itch) with scratch marks may be associated with chronic kidney disease and obstructive jaundice because toxins are deposited in the skin.

3. **Look for rashes**. Tender, raised ulcerated areas on the legs (**pyoderma gangrenosum**) are an important but uncommon sign of inflammatory bowel disease.
4. Look for the neurological signs of alcoholism (e.g. a coarse tremor) or evidence of thiamine deficiency (peripheral neuropathy or memory loss; p. 188).

The genitourinary system

The genitourinary system assessment also involves a careful abdominal examination. The sequence is set out below.

The genitourinary system assessment sequence

1. Presenting symptoms (e.g. changes in the urine or symptoms during micturition [pain, poor stream, nocturia], abdominal or flank pain, fever, malaise)
2. Detailed questions about presenting symptoms (SOCRATES)
3. Questions about previous urinary problems and procedures or operations, known abnormalities of kidney function, risk factors for kidney disease (e.g. hypertension, diabetes mellitus)
4. History of dialysis or renal transplantation
5. Blood pressure, and examination for peripheral signs of chronic kidney disease or dialysis
6. Examination of the abdomen: renal masses, peritoneal dialysis fluid
7. Examination of the genitals, if appropriate, assessment for oedema, and testing of the urine
8. Provisional and differential diagnosis

PRESENTING SYMPTOMS (see Box 6.4)

1. Patients may present with urinary tract symptoms (changes in the urine or in micturition) or abdominal or flank pain.

T&O'C examination hint box

Many patients with kidney disease have no symptoms but are found to be hypertensive or to have abnormalities on routine urinalysis or serum biochemistry.

Box 6.4
The genitourinary history: presenting symptoms

Major symptoms
Change in appearance of urine (e.g. haematuria—red discolouration)
Change in urine volume or stream
Polyuria (an increase in the volume of urine)
Nocturia (getting up to pass urine during the night)
Oliguria (reduced urine output: <400 mL/day)
Anuria (little or no urine output: <50 mL/day)
Symptoms of prostatic enlargement
- Decrease in stream size
- Hesitancy
- Dribbling
- Urine retention
- Urinary frequency
- Urinary urgency (the need to pass urine without delay)
Incontinence of urine (stress incontinence, e.g. on coughing; urge incontinence)
Double voiding (incomplete bladder emptying)
Renal colic
Symptoms of urinary infection
- Dysuria (painful micturition), frequency (the need to pass small amounts of urine frequently), urgency, fever, loin pain
Urethral discharge
Symptoms suggestive of chronic kidney disease (uraemia)
- Oliguria, nocturia, polyuria
- Anorexia, a metallic taste, vomiting, fatigue, hiccups, insomnia
- Itch, bruising, oedema
Erectile dysfunction
Loss of libido
Infertility
Urethral or vaginal discharge
Genital rash

2. Ask about:
   - a change in the appearance of the urine
   - symptoms of urinary obstruction (e.g. hesitancy, decrease in the size of the stream, terminal dribbling)
   - urinary incontinence.
3. Ask about **symptoms of chronic kidney disease**; these are not specific but can include:
   - nocturia
   - anorexia
   - vomiting

- fatigue
- hiccups
- insomnia
- pruritus.

4. Obtain a **menstrual history** from females (including the date of menarche and the regularity of the menstrual cycle). Ask about:
   - dysmenorrhoea (painful menstruation)
   - menorrhagia (abnormally heavy periods)
   - vaginal discharge
   - the number of pregnancies and births
   - complications of pregnancy and childbirth (e.g. hypertension)
   - contraceptive methods.

PAST HISTORY

Find out about:
- recurrent urinary tract infections or calculi
- renal surgery
- previous detection of proteinuria or microscopic haematuria
- a diagnosis of diabetes mellitus, gout or hypertension
- performance of a renal biopsy (this is usually memorable).

SOCIAL HISTORY

Ask about any social problems, and in renal failure patients ask how the patient has coped and is coping with a serious chronic illness.

TREATMENT

1. Take a detailed drug history.
2. Find out whether the patient is undergoing dialysis[3] and whether this is haemodialysis or peritoneal dialysis.
3. Find out whether the patient has had a renal transplant. If so, ask about:
   - how well the graft is working (many patients know their current creatinine and e-GFR [estimated glomerular filtration rate])

---

3 Sometimes rather grandly and not altogether accurately called *renal replacement therapy.*

- problems with rejection and how these were managed (e.g. renal biopsy and increase in drug treatment)
- drug treatment and side effects
- problems with osteoporosis.

FAMILY HISTORY

Ask particularly about polycystic kidney disease, diabetes mellitus and hypertension in the family.

Examination of the genitourinary system

This is not part of the routine examination but should be a targeted evaluation based on the history.

1. Assess the **state of hydration** in all patients with suspected renal (or gastrointestinal) disease, including testing skin turgor, checking for tachycardia and measuring the blood pressure for postural hypotension. Dehydration can be a cause of acute renal failure, while overhydration can result from intravenous infusions of fluid when attempts are made to correct acute renal failure.

2. As in the gastrointestinal examination, you can start with the hands and progress to the abdomen and genitalia as indicated. Note the general signs of end-stage chronic kidney disease.

HANDS AND ARMS

1. Look at the **nails** for *white nails* (low albumin states, including leakage from the kidneys) and *half-and-half nails* (distal nail brown–red, proximal nail pink–white) from chronic kidney disease.

2. Palmar crease pallor suggests anaemia (anaemia is common in chronic kidney disease).

3. Palpate the wrists for surgically created **arteriovenous fistulae** or **shunts** used for haemodialysis access. There is a longitudinal swelling and a palpable, continuous thrill present over a fistula.

4. You may see bruising, subcutaneous nodules or scratch marks in chronic kidney disease.

5. Take the blood pressure with the patient lying down and standing. It may be high in chronic kidney disease and low if there is dehydration causing acute renal failure.

NECK AND CHEST

1. Examine the jugular venous pressure to assess intravascular volume status—in chronic kidney disease the patient may be volume overloaded.
2. Examine the heart and lungs for signs of cardiac failure, pericarditis and pulmonary oedema, which can all occur in chronic kidney disease.

ABDOMEN

1. Do a complete examination.
2. Look for scars:
   - Nephrectomy scars are often more posterior than might be expected; they usually lie in the flank as far posterior as the erector spinae muscle group.
   - Renal transplant scars are usually found in the right or left lower abdomen (iliac fossae) and a **transplanted kidney** may be visible as a bulge under the scar.
   - Previous peritoneal dialysis results in small scars from catheter placement in the peritoneal cavity; these are situated on the lower abdomen at or near the mid-line.
3. Focus on palpating the kidneys (e.g. enlarged in polycystic kidney disease). A transplanted kidney may be felt under a scar. While ballotting for the kidney, note any tenderness over the renal angle.
4. Auscultate for a renal bruit (listen above the umbilicus 2 cm to the left or right of the mid-line).
5. A rectal examination in men to feel for prostastomegaly is relevant, as a large prostate may cause urinary obstruction.

MALE GENITALIA

1. Inspect the scrotum for size and skin changes (e.g. ulceration).

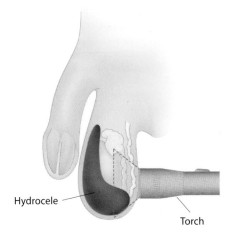

Figure 6.15 Transillumination of the testes.

2. (Wearing gloves) Palpate the scrotum for the **testes**. Feel each testis rather gently and note the size, regularity and firmness.
3. The **spermatic cord** is palpable as it enters the scrotum: the **epididymis** on top of each testis is also usually palpable.
4. There may be a mass in the scrotum separate from the testes. If it is not possible to find the upper limit of this mass, it must have descended into the testis from above and is probably an inguinal hernia.
5. A mass wholly within the testis should be tested for transillumination (see Fig 6.15) with a torch.
6. A hydrocele is confined to the scrotum, will usually light up in an impressive manner, and the testis and epididymis are not palpable.
7. Examine the **penis** if indicated. Inspect, looking for:
   - urethral discharge
   - rash
   - inflammation
   - a mass.
8. Next palpate the glans penis through the foreskin, retract the foreskin (which will not be possible if the patient has phimosis) and palpate the inguinal glands.

T&O'C examination hint box

Bilateral **testicular atrophy** occurs in chronic liver disease (e.g. alcoholic liver disease, haemochromatosis) rather than local testicular disease.

T&O'C examination hint box

If there is a lump in the scrotum, see if you can feel above it; you cannot get above a hernia. The upper end of a hydrocele is palpable in the inguinal canal, so you can get above a hydrocele in the inguinal canal but not a hernia.

OTHER SIGNS

1. Assess for peripheral oedema, sacral oedema and rashes.
2. Look in the fundi for evidence of retinal findings suggestive of hypertension (p. 234) or diabetes mellitus (a common cause of chronic kidney disease; p. 316).
3. A **urinalysis** provides initial bedside evidence of possible renal disease. The urine can be tested with a dipstick for certain abnormalities. Colour changes on the stick will indicate the pH, protein (proteinuria), sugar (diabetes mellitus), nitrites (possible infection) and red blood cells (haematuria).

The haematological system

The haematological examination begins with a search for peripheral signs and extends to an abdominal examination. Again, this is not routine but a targeted assessment based on the history. The suggested sequence is set out below.

The haematological system assessment sequence

1. Presenting symptoms (e.g. lethargy, dyspnoea, pallor, easy bruising, abdominal pain, lymph node enlargement)
2. Detailed questions about presenting symptoms (SOCRATES)
3. Questions about previous haematological problems and procedures, known blood test results
4. Examination for peripheral signs of haematological disease
5. Examination of all lymph node groups
6. Examination of the abdomen: focus on hepatosplenomegaly
7. Provisional and differential diagnosis

PRESENTING SYMPTOMS (see Box 6.5)

1. Patients may present with symptoms of anaemia (lethargy, palpitations, dyspnoea on exertion or angina).
2. Alternatively, the presenting symptoms may be of the condition leading to anaemia or of the causes of anaemia, such as rectal bleeding or the bowel symptoms of malabsorption.
3. The patient who complains of lymph node enlargement should be asked about night sweats and weight loss (e.g. lymphoma).
4. Recurrent infection with fevers may be the first symptom of a disorder of the immune system or of neutropenia.
5. Take a detailed history from patients who easily bruise or bleed, including questions about postoperative bleeding.
   - If bleeding after trauma is immediate, this suggests a platelet problem.
   - If bleeding occurs after a delay, a clotting factor problem is more likely.

Box 6.5
The haematological history: presenting symptoms

Major symptoms
Symptoms of anaemia: weakness, tiredness, dyspnoea, fatigue, postural dizziness
Bleeding (menstrual, gastrointestinal)
Easy bruising
Thrombotic tendency (e.g. repeated deep venous thrombosis in the legs)
Recurrent infection, fever
Jaundice
Lymph gland enlargement
Bone pain
Paraesthesias (e.g. vitamin B_{12} deficiency)
Skin rash
Weight loss
Night sweats

PAST HISTORY

1. Ask about systemic disease and previous gastric surgery as causes of anaemia.

2. Ask whether the patient has been refused as a blood donor and, if so, why.

TREATMENT

1. Find out about the use of:
   - iron supplements
   - vitamin B_{12} injections
   - NSAIDs
   - anticoagulants
2. Also ask about any chemotherapy, previous blood transfusions or therapeutic venesections (blood taken to remove iron from the body).

FAMILY HISTORY

There may be a family history of:
- thalassaemia
- haemolytic anaemia (or jaundice)
- haemophilia
- von Willebrand's disease
- factor V Leiden (a cause of increased clotting risk) (thrombophilia).

Haematopoeitic examination

Just as in the gastrointestinal system, you can start with the hands. You must examine the lymph nodes in all regions and the abdomen.

HANDS AND ARMS

1. Look for signs of anaemia.
2. Inspect the nails. Look for **koilonychia**—dry, brittle, ridged, spoon-shaped nails sometimes due to severe iron-deficiency anaemia (see Table 3.2); this is now rare.
3. Look for bruising and petechiae. If petechiae are raised (palpable petechiae), consider a vasculitis.
4. Examine *all* of the **lymph node groups on both sides** (arms, axillae, neck).
   - To examine the **epitrochlear lymph nodes**, place the palm of your left hand under the patient's right elbow. Your thumb can then be placed over the node that is

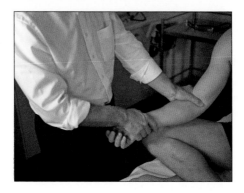

Figure 6.16 Feeling for the epitrochlear lymph node.

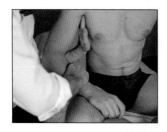
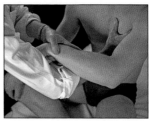

Figure 6.17 Palpating the axillary lymph nodes.

proximal and slightly anterior to the medial epicondyle (see Fig 6.16). Repeat with your right hand for the other side.

- The **axillary lymph nodes** are palpated by raising the patient's arm and, using your left hand for the right side, pushing your fingers as high as possible into the axilla. The patient's arm is then brought down to rest on your forearm. The opposite is done for the other side (see Fig 6.17). There are five main groups of axillary nodes: (1) central; (2) lateral (above and lateral); (3) pectoral (medial); (4) infraclavicular; and (5) subscapular (most inferior). An effort should be made to feel for nodes in each of these areas of the axilla (see Fig 6.18).

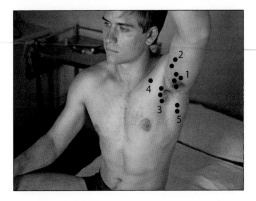

Figure 6.18   The axillary lymph nodes. 1 = central,
2 = lateral, 3 = pectoral, 4 = infraclavicular, 5 = subscapular.

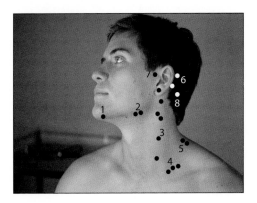

Figure 6.19   Cervical and supraclavicular lymph node groups.
1 = submental, 2 = submandibular, 3 = jugular chain, 4 = supraclavicular,
5 = posterior triangle, 6 = postauricular, 7 = preauricular, 8 = occipital.

- Examine the **cervical and supraclavicular lymph nodes** from behind (preferred) or in front. There are eight groups: (1) submental; (2) submandibular; (3) jugular chain; (4) supraclavicular; (5) posterior triangle; (6) postauricular; (7) preauricular; and (8) occipital. Attempt to identify each group of nodes with your fingers (see Fig 6.19).

- First palpate the **submental** node, which lies directly under the chin, then the **submandibular** nodes, which are below the angle of the jaw.
- Next palpate the **jugular chain**, which lies anterior to the sternomastoid muscle, and then the **posterior triangle** nodes, which are posterior to the sternocleidomastoid muscle.
- Palpate the **occipital** region for occipital nodes and then move to the **postauricular** node behind the ear and the **preauricular** node in front of the ear.
- With the patient's shoulders slightly shrugged, feel in the supraclavicular fossa and at the base of the sternocleidomastoid muscle for the **supraclavicular** nodes.

FACE

1. Look for signs of jaundice or anaemia. Look in the mouth for gum hypertrophy (from leukaemia) or bleeding.
2. Look in the fundi (p. 233). Look for engorged retinal vessels and papilloedema. This can occur in diseases such as macroglobulinaemia which increase blood viscosity. Haemorrhages may occur with severe thrombocytopenia, especially when it is associated with anaemia.

ABDOMEN

You need to do a careful abdominal examination focusing on the liver and spleen, which can both be enlarged by lymphoma or leukaemia.

INGUINAL LYMPH NODES

After informing the patient, palpate over the inguinal region. Note any lymph nodes. There are two groups:
- one along the inguinal ligament
- the other along the femoral vessels.

Small (<1 cm diameter), firm, mobile nodes are commonly found in healthy people.

SPINE

Tap over the spine for bony tenderness (suggesting bone marrow infiltration).

LEGS

1. Look for leg ulcers, which can occur in a number of blood diseases such as sickle cell anaemia. Vitamin B_{12} deficiency can cause anaemia and signs of peripheral neuropathy (p. 318).

2. Popliteal nodes are not routinely felt for as they are rarely palpable.

T&O'C examination hint box: Characteristics of lymph nodes

During palpation of the lymph nodes the following features must be considered.

Site
Palpable nodes may be localised to one region (e.g. local infection, early lymphoma) or generalised (e.g. late lymphoma). The palpable lymph node areas are:
- epitrochlear
- axillary
- cervical (includes occipital and supraclavicular)
- para-aortic (rarely palpable) in the abdomen
- inguinal
- popliteal (behind the knee).

Size
Large nodes are usually abnormal (>1 cm).

Consistency
- Hard nodes suggest carcinoma deposits.
- Soft nodes may be normal.
- Rubbery nodes may be due to lymphoma.

Tenderness
This implies infection or acute inflammation.

Fixation
Nodes that are fixed to underlying structures are more likely to be infiltrated by carcinoma than mobile nodes.

Overlying skin
Inflammation of the overlying skin suggests infection, and tethering to the overlying skin suggests carcinoma.

You need to develop a system to examine the patient from whose history you suspect or are worried about a malignancy. A suggested approach is as follows.

Examining the patient with suspected malignancy
1. Palpate all draining lymph nodes.
2. Examine all remaining lymph node groups.
3. Examine the abdomen, particularly for hepatomegaly and ascites.
4. Examine the lungs.
5. Examine the breasts.
6. Examine the skin and nails (e.g. for melanoma).
7. Perform a rectal examination and pelvic examination to complete the evaluation.
8. Feel the testes.

The abdomen OSCE: hints panel

1. This man has noticed that his sclerae have turned yellow. Take a history from him.
   (a) This is likely to be jaundice (which should be obvious on inspection). Ask him the following:
       (i) Have you noticed a change in the colour of your skin and the whites of your eyes?
       (ii) How long has it been present? Is it getting better or worse? Has it happened before?
       (iii) Are you itchy?
       (iv) Has the colour of your urine or stools changed? (Dark urine and pale stools in obstructive jaundice)
       (v) Have you lost weight? (e.g. malignancy involving the liver or pancreas)
       (vi) Do you have any abdominal pain? (Ask about the symptoms of biliary pain)
       (vii) Does your abdomen swell up (ascites)? Do you develop leg swelling (oedema)?
       (viii) Have you ever vomited blood or passed black stools? (Haematemesis and melaena—may be from bleeding oesophageal varices)
       (ix) Have you ever had hepatitis? Have you travelled overseas? (Infection hepatitis)
       (x) Have you had fatigue, nausea, anorexia, myalgias, bruising?
       (xi) Are you a diabetic? (Haemochromatosis)
       (xii) Do you now drink, or have you in the past drunk, large amounts of alcohol?

       (xiii) Do you suffer any memory loss or confusion? (Hepatic encephalopathy)

       (xiv) Have you had a liver biopsy? Do you know what is wrong with your liver? (Probe for alcohol abuse)

   (b) Does the patient have any history of blood transfusions, drug use, tattoos or body piercing (e.g. hepatitis C or B)?

   (c) Take the sexual history.

   (d) Take the medication history (drug-induced hepatitis).

   (e) Check whether there is a family history of liver problems.

   (f) Synthesise and present your findings.

2. This man has been diagnosed as having liver failure. Please examine his abdomen. (Wash your hands)

   (a) Ask the patient's permission to examine his abdomen and ask him to lie flat with his abdomen exposed from the lower ribs to the symphysis pubis.

   (b) While the patient is undressing, stand back to look for obvious signs of chronic liver disease.

   (c) Ask whether any part of his abdomen is tender and to let you know if any part of the examination is uncomfortable.

   (d) Examine the abdomen systematically (inspect, palpate, percuss, auscultate). Assess particularly for ascites and hepatosplenomegaly.

   (e) Ask whether you may examine other regions. Note any jaundice or scleral pallor (anaemia).

   (f) Look for spider naevi and gynaecomastia on the chest wall (signs of chronic liver disease).

   (g) Look for finger clubbing, leuconychia and palmar erythema (signs of chronic liver disease).

   (h) Test for a liver flap and fetor hepaticus, and assess orientation and mental state (liver failure).

   (i) Synthesise and present your findings.

3. Please examine this man's abdomen. He has a family history of renal impairment and hypertension. (Wash your hands)

   (a) Ask the patient's permission to examine his abdomen and ask him to lie flat with his abdomen exposed from the lower ribs to the symphysis pubis.

   (b) Look for abdominal distension.

   (c) Ask about areas of tenderness.

   (d) Examine the abdomen, paying particular attention to palpation of the kidneys since a possible diagnosis is polycystic kidneys.

   (e) Attempt to outline the size of the kidneys and detect the characteristic cystic shape.

   (f) Ballott the kidneys and demonstrate that you can get above them (i.e. that there is renal enlargement, not hepatosplenomegaly).

   (g) Assess the liver and spleen (may also be polycystic).

   (h) Take the blood pressure.

   (i) Synthesise and present your findings.

4. This woman has a lymphoma. Please examine her abdomen. (Wash your hands)
   (a) Ask the patient's permission to examine her abdomen and ask her to lie flat with her abdomen exposed from the lower ribs to the symphysis pubis.
   (b) While the patient is undressing, look for wasting, abdominal distension and surgical scars.
   (c) Ask about tenderness or discomfort.
   (d) Examine her abdomen. Pay particular attention to the size of the liver and spleen, and palpate for enlarged abdominal lymph nodes.
   (e) Examine all the other lymph node groups, starting with the inguinal nodes.
   (f) Ask whether you have time to examine the chest.
   (g) Synthesise and present your findings.

5. This man has a hernia in the groin. Please examine him. (Wash your hands and don gloves)
   (a) Explain to the patient what you want to do and ask his permission.
   (b) Ask him to stand in front of you and remove his underpants.
   (c) Inspect the groin for lumps on both sides.
   (d) Try to decide whether the lump is an inguinal hernia or a femoral hernia by palpation of its position.
   (e) Ask the patient to cough and feel for a cough impulse.
   (f) Palpate. Find your landmarks. Gently push the lump back into the abdomen. Is it reducible?
   (g) Invaginate the scrotum gently and feel for the external ring and an impulse as the patient coughs, if you suspect an inguinal hernia.
   (h) Note the number of testes in the scrotum.
   (i) Lay him down and inspect and palpate the groin.
   (j) Synthesise and present your findings.

6. This woman has found a lump in her neck. Please examine her lymph nodes. (Wash your hands)
   (a) Ask the patient to remove her shirt and sit up over the edge of the bed.
   (b) Stand back to look for wasting or obvious scars or abdominal distension.
   (c) Examine the cervical (including the supraclavicular) nodes with her in this position, then examine the axillary and epitrochlear nodes. Keep in mind the characteristics of different lymph node abnormalities.
   (d) Next lay the patient flat and expose the abdomen.
   (e) Feel for inguinal nodes, for splenomegaly and for hepatomegaly.
   (f) If a group of nodes is abnormal, consider their area of drainage and ask to examine that region. If many groups are enlarged, consider a lymphoma as the cause.
   (g) Synthesise and present your findings.

T&O'C examination essentials

The abdominal history and examination

1. Eliciting the individual symptoms and the pattern of presentation will often lead to the correct diagnosis.

2. When examining the abdomen, it is important to position the patient flat. While palpating, consider the underlying organs that are present when abnormalities are detected.

3. If an abdominal mass is found, characterise it carefully. Assess whether the liver, spleen and kidneys are palpable.

4. A left upper quadrant mass may be a spleen or a kidney. Remember that one cannot get above the spleen and that the spleen is not ballottable.

5. An inguinal hernia bulges above the crease of the groin, whereas a femoral hernia bulges into the groin crease at its medial end.

7

Neurology

The whole art of medicine is in observation.

Sir William Osler (1849–1919)

Neurological history taking and examination require an approach that is very systematic and thorough. Only by this means can the symptoms and signs be assembled in a way that will enable a sensible neurological diagnosis.

The neurological system assessment sequence

1. Presenting symptoms (e.g. headache, syncope, dizziness, sensory changes, motor weakness, balance problems)
2. Detailed questions about the presenting symptoms and especially their time course (SOCRATES)
3. Questions about previous neurological problems and risk factors (e.g. family history, hypertension, medications), results of precious investigations and handedness
4. General examination for orientation.
5. Examination of the cranial nerves (including fundi)
6. Examination of the motor system and reflexes (including gait)
7. Sensory system examination, directed by the history and other examination findings
8. Provisional and differential diagnosis

The neurological history

PRESENTING SYMPTOMS (see Box 7.1)

The **temporal course of a neurological illness** usually gives important information about the underlying aetiology:

- An acute onset of symptoms suggests a vascular problem.
- A subacute onset suggests an inflammatory disorder.
- A more chronic symptom course suggests that the underlying disorder may be related to either a tumour or a degenerative process.

Box 7.1
Neurological history

Presenting symptoms
Headache
Facial pain
Back or neck pain
Fits, faints or funny turns
Vertigo or dizziness
Disturbances of vision, hearing or smell
Disturbances of gait
Loss of or disturbed sensation, or weakness in a limb or limbs
Disturbances of sphincter control (bladder, bowels)
Involuntary movements or tremor
Speech and swallowing disturbance
Altered cognition (see Ch 13)

Risk factors for cerebrovascular disease
Hypertension
Smoking
Diabetes mellitus
Hyperlipidaemia
Atrial fibrillation, bacterial endocarditis, valvular heart disease
Bleeding disorders, anticoagulant drugs, thrombophilic disorders
Family history of stroke

T&O'C examination hint box

The neurological examination is one of the most difficult to perform while being watched. Only constant practice will enable students to look competent with the various aspects of this examination when they are under the pressure of an OSCE or short case examination.

Metabolic or toxic disorders may present with any of these patterns. Episodic or recurrent symptoms may be vascular (e.g. transient ischaemic attacks or migraines), due to vestibular disease, or due to seizures.

A judgement must also be made as to whether the disease process is **localised** or **diffuse**, and what levels of the nervous system are involved.

Headache and facial pain

Headache is a common and difficult symptom but the diagnosis may be clear once the pattern has been determined.

- **Tension-type headache** may be episodic or chronic, commonly bilateral, and occurs over the frontal, occipital or temporal areas. It may be described as a sensation of tightness. These headaches last for hours, recur often and lack the specific features of other headaches. This is the most common type.
- **Classical migraine** is usually a unilateral headache preceded by an aura (e.g. flashing lights) and is commonly associated with photophobia (light intolerance). It is often of incapacitating severity and associated with nausea and vomiting. **Common migraine** is a similar headache without the other neurological symptoms and is much more common.
- **Cluster headache** is a severe, steady boring pain behind or over one eye lasting 15 minutes to 2 hours, associated with lacrimation, rhinorrhoea and flushing of the forehead. It tends to occur at the same time each day, often at night.
- **Headache due to cervical spondylosis** occurs over the occiput that is associated with neck pain.
- **Headache caused by raised intracranial pressure** is generalised and worse in the morning. It may be associated with drowsiness or vomiting and progressive neurological deficits.
- **Meningitis headache** is generalised headache and associated with photophobia, fever and a stiff neck.
- **Temporal arteritis headache** is persistent and felt over the temporal area. There is associated tenderness over the temporal artery. There may be jaw claudication (pain on eating or talking) as well as acute visual loss.

- **Acute sinusitis headache** is associated with pain or fullness behind the eyes or over the cheeks or forehead (over the inflamed sinuses).
- **Subarachnoid haemorrhage headache** is dramatic, severe and usually of instantaneous onset.

Faints and fits

Transient loss of consciousness may have a neurological cause, but cardiac arrhythmias and metabolic diseases are other possible explanations. The following should be considered.

- **Syncope** due to a simple faint is the most common cause of loss of consciousness. The episode is usually very brief and is often preceded by pallor, sweating (clamminess), nausea and dizziness (in this case a feeling of impending loss of consciousness). If the degree of cerebral hypoperfusion is severe, there may be a few clonic jerks or a brief tonic spasm ('convulsive syncope'). There tends to be minimal confusion following the episode.
- A **seizure (epilepsy)** is characterised by an abrupt loss of consciousness. It may be preceded by an aura—an abnormal sensation (e.g. a hallucination involving one of the senses, or altered cognition such as a sense of deja vu). Bystanders may have observed tonic (sustained contraction of the muscles for 20–30 seconds) and clonic (violent rhythmical) movements. Patients who have had a major seizure may sleep for a period after the episode and may wake to find that they have bitten their tongue and been incontinent.
- **Transient ischaemic attacks** can affect the brainstem. These may rarely cause loss of consciousness without warning.
- **Hypoglycaemia** usually occurs in diabetic patients on insulin or taking oral hypoglycaemic drugs. These patients may feel anxious and sweaty and notice a fast heart rate before unconsciousness occurs—these are autonomic nervous system responses to hypoglycaemia.
- **Hysteria** may cause bizarre attacks of apparent loss of consciousness.[1]

---

1 Hysteria is an old term referring to a presumed psychogenic condition. This is not the same as malingering. Hysterical patients are not pretending.

Vertigo and dizziness

In true **vertigo**, there is actually a sense of motion. The world seems to turn around. There is a feeling of loss of balance rather than of impending syncope. It can be caused by vestibular disease (acute labyrinthitis, benign positional vertigo or Ménière's disease) or cerebellar disease (such as that caused by alcohol, anticonvulsants, multiple sclerosis, vascular lesions or tumour).

Dizziness can be a feeling of impending unconsciousness or merely of momentary unsteadiness.

T&O'C examination hint box

It is not enough to accept a patient's description of the problem as 'dizziness'. Careful questioning is required to understand what the feeling actually is and to impress the examiners.

T&O'C examination hint box

Categories of dizziness
- **Vertigo:** a false sense of motion, often with a sensation of the world or the patient's head spinning.
- **Disequilibrium:** a feeling of loss of balance (may be a result of cerebellar disease [Romberg's sign negative] or peripheral neuropathy [Romberg's sign positive]).
- **Presyncope:** a feeling of impending loss of consciousness.
- **Light-headedness:** vague symptoms that may include a feeling of de-realisation or disconnection with the surroundings.

Disturbances of vision, hearing or smell

These symptoms may reflect a cranial nerve lesion. Ask about:
- double vision (diplopia)
- blurred vision
- loss of vision (amblyopia)
- light intolerance (photophobia)
- loss of hearing in one or both ears
- ringing in the ears (tinnitus).

Disturbances of gait

Many neurological conditions can make walking difficult.

- **Cerebellar disease** makes walking unsteady and uncertain.
- **Hemiplegia** after a stroke makes walking difficult because of an increase in tone and loss of power in the affected leg.
- A **peripheral neuropathy** or spinal cord disease may alter position sense in the legs. Parkinson's disease causes a characteristic shuffling gait.
- **Hysteria** can present with a bizarrely abnormal gait.
- Walking may also be abnormal when **orthopaedic or rheumatological disease** affects the lower limbs or spine.

Disturbed sensation or weakness in the limbs

Pins and needles in the hands or feet more often indicates nerve entrapment or a peripheral neuropathy but can result from sensory pathway involvement at any level.

Limb weakness may be due to cerebral, spinal cord (including anterior horn cell), nerve root, peripheral nerve, neuromuscular junction or muscle disease. Distinguishing between an upper and a lower motor neuron lesion is important (see box on p. 200).

Autonomic symptoms

Ask about bladder or bowel incontinence, erectile dysfunction (in men) and postural dizziness, all of which may be symptoms of autonomic neuropathy.

Tremor and involuntary movements

Tremors are fine involuntary repetitive movements.

- **Action tremors** are worse when a voluntary movement is attempted. These include an enhanced physiological tremor, as may occur in essential tremors, anxiety and thyrotoxicosis.
- **Intention** (or **target seeking**) **tremors** become worse as the limb gets closer to the object reached for and are due to cerebellar disease.
- Parkinson's disease may present with a **resting tremor** (characteristically a 'pill rolling' tremor).
- **Chorea** means irregular jerky movements.

PAST MEDICAL HISTORY

Enquire about a past history of:

- meningitis or encephalitis
- head or spinal injuries and epilepsy
- risk factors for human immunodeficiency virus (HIV) infection or syphilis, which may have nervous system involvement
- use of anticonvulsant drugs, the contraceptive pill, antihypertensive agents, chemotherapeutic agents, anti-Parkinsonian drugs, steroids, anticoagulants and anti-platelet agents, which may be used for neurological conditions or may have neurological effects.

Also ask about risk factors that may predispose to the development of cerebrovascular disease (see Box 7.1).

SOCIAL HISTORY

As smoking predisposes to cerebrovascular disease, the smoking history is relevant. It is also useful to ask about occupation and exposure to toxins (e.g. heavy metals, pesticides). Alcohol intake can result in a number of neurological diseases, such as cerebellar degeneration, short-term memory impairment and peripheral neuropathy.

FAMILY HISTORY

Any history of neurological or mental disease should be documented.

Neurological examination sequence

The neurological examination is complicated but rewarding. Adequate interpretation of neurological signs requires an understanding of basic neuroanatomy. The following components must be systematically assessed.

1. **General.** This includes examination for the level of consciousness (see Ch 14), orientation, handedness ('Are you right- or left-handed?') and the presence of neck stiffness, and the assessment of speech and the higher centres.
2. **Cranial nerves.** Examine cranial nerves II (including the fundi) to XII. The first (olfactory) nerve is often omitted

but anosmia (absence of ability to smell) may be the only sign of a frontal meningioma.

3. **Upper limbs.** Assessment involves:
   - **motor system:** inspection, tone, power, reflexes and coordination
   - **sensory system:** pain (pin-prick) sensation, light touch, proprioception (position sense) and vibration sense.
4. **Lower limbs.** Assess as for the upper limbs (motor and sensory systems) but include an assessment of walking (gait).
5. **Skull and spine.** Assess for local disease (scars, signs of injury, lumps), if relevant.
6. **Carotid arteries.** Auscultate both sides for bruits. There may be no bruit with severe carotid stenosis (>90% blockage). It may not be possible to diagnose a separate carotid bruit in patients with aortic stenosis.

GENERAL

Neck stiffness and Kernig's sign

This examination is absolutely essential for any febrile or acutely ill patient, or for anyone with altered mental status. See also Chapter 14.

1. Slip one hand under the patient's head and attempt to gently flex the head so that the patient's chin touches the chest (see Fig 7.1).

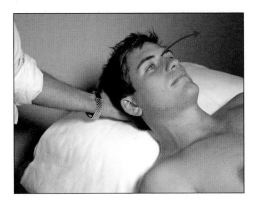

Figure 7.1   Testing for neck stiffness.

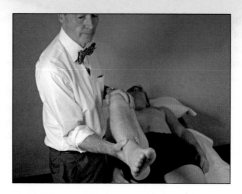

Figure 7.2 Testing for Kernig's sign (legs).

2. Resistance due to painful spasm of the extensor muscles of the neck will occur if the meninges are inflamed.
3. Next, flex the patient's hip and then attempt to straighten the patient's knee. Painful spasm of the hamstrings will occur if there is inflammation around the lumbar spinal roots—**Kernig's sign** (see Fig 7.2).

Handedness, orientation, speech and higher centres

1. Ask the patient whether he or she is right- or left-handed (to help determine the likely dominant hemisphere, which is in the left brain in most right-handed people).
2. As a screening assessment, ask for the patient's name, present location and the date. This tests **orientation** in person, place and time. These tests are part of the mental state examination.
3. Next ask the patient to name an object pointed at,[2] then to point to a named object in the room. This screens for dysphasia:
   - **Receptive dysphasia** is an inability to understand speech.
   - **Expressive dysphasia** is an inability to answer appropriately.
   - **Nominal dysphasia** is an inability to name objects.

---

2 Remember that you may not be the only one to attempt a joke. Patients may attempt to conceal their nominal aphasia by using a different word as if joking—for example, if asked to name the consultant's watch, the patient may say 'expensive'.

- **Conductive dysphasia** is an inability to repeat speech (see T&OC examination essentials box below).
4. **Dysarthria** is a problem with the mechanical production of speech. Ask the patient to say 'West Register Street' or 'British Constitution'. This is a test for cerebellar dysfunction and its effect on speech. Cerebellar disease (and acute alcoholic intoxication) causes slurring and staccato speech.
5. **Dysphonia** refers to impaired sound production from the larynx. Ask the patient to say 'Aaah' and to cough.

T&O'C examination essentials

Assessment of a patient with dysphasia
- **Wernicke's area** in the superior posterior **temporal lobe** of the dominant cerebral hemisphere comprehends speech. A lesion here causes **receptive (sensory) dysphasia**.
- **Broca's area** in the inferior **frontal lobe** of the dominant cerebral hemisphere controls language expression. A lesion here causes **expressive (motor) dysphasia.**
- The **arcuate fasciculus** connects Wernicke's and Broca's areas. A lesion here causes **conduction dysphasia**.

Fluent speech (receptive or conductive dysphasia)
1. *Naming objects.* Patients with conductive and receptive dysphasia will name objects poorly. In nominal dysphasia, this is the only abnormality (dominant posterior temporoparietal lesion).
2. *Repetition.* Patients with conductive and receptive dysphasia have difficult repeating words or phrases.
3. *Comprehension.* Patients with receptive dysphasia cannot follow commands (verbal or written). In conductive dysphasia commands can be followed.

Non-fluent speech (expressive dysphasia)
1. *Naming objects.* This is absent or poor but may be better than spontaneous speech.
2. *Repetition.* This may be possible with great effort. Phrase repetition (e.g. 'No ifs, ands or buts') is poor.
3. *Comprehension.* This is relatively normal, and written and verbal commands can be followed.
4. *Reading.* Patients may have dyslexia.
5. *Writing.* Dysgraphia may be present.
6. *Look for hemiparesis* (upper motor neuron weakness on one side). The arm is more affected than the leg.

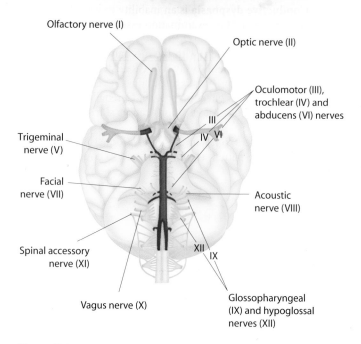

Figure 7.3 The location of the cranial nerves.

CRANIAL NERVES

The patient should be sat over the edge of the bed if possible. Begin with a general inspection of the head and neck. Look for **craniotomy** scars, which suggest previous surgery that has required opening of the skull. Then examine the cranial nerves in roughly the order of their number (see Fig 7.3). The use of a systematic approach is the only way to be sure nothing important is left out.

The first (olfactory) nerve

Testing is not performed routinely but is required if there is suspected loss of smell (anosmia). Each nostril is tested separately using non-pungent substances in a series of sample bottles. The patient sniffs these delicately and should be able to identify common smells, such as coffee and vanilla. An alcohol wipe is enough for a simple test of smell.

The second (optic) nerve (see also Ch 8)

1. Always test **visual acuity** with the patient wearing his or her reading spectacles, if required.
   - Test each eye separately, while the other is covered with a small card.
   - Ask the patient to read letters on a chart. The standard chart is read reflected in a mirror from 3 m away (effectively 6 m). The ability to read the letters normally visible at this distance is called 6/6 vision. The ability to read only larger letters normally visible at 60 m is called 6/60 vision. A hand-held chart can be carried and used as an alternative.
   - Patients with poor visual acuity may only be able to distinguish hand movements or light and dark.
2. Examine the **visual fields**. One method involves confrontation with a red-topped hatpin. In this examination the patient's field of vision is compared with yours (see Fig 7.4a). Your head should be level with the patient's head.
   - Slowly bring the pin into each quadrant diagonally. When the pin is brought into your visual field and the patient's, it should become visible to both of you at the same point.
   - You must watch for the pin and also watch the patient's eye to ensure that it remains looking straight ahead. Patients are often tempted to look towards the pin.

   A number of visual field defects can be detected, as shown in Figure 7.4b.

   If visual acuity is poor, the fields are mapped using the fingers instead of a pin. Ask the patient to say when your first and second fingers become visible as they are brought into the quadrants of the visual fields. With practice the fields can be mapped with your fingers—this is how ophthalmologists perform the test.
3. Examine the **fundi** (p. 233).

T&O'C examination hint box

When asking the patient to cover one eye with the hand, tell the patient to use the palm of the hand rather than the fingers. It is usually possible to see through the fingers and vision is therefore not occluded completely.

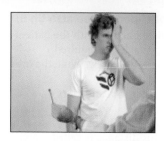

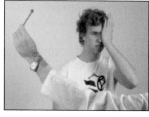

(a)

1	**Tunnel vision:** concentric diminution (e.g. glaucoma, papilloedema)	
2	**Enlarged blind spot:** optic nerve head enlargement	
3	**Central scotomata:** optic nerve head to chiasmal lesion (e.g. demyelination, toxic, vascular, nutritional)	
4	**Unilateral field loss:** optic nerve lesion (e.g. vascular, tumour)	
5	**Bitemporal hemianopia:** optic chiasm lesion (e.g. pituitary tumour, sella meningioma)	
6	**Homonymous hemianopia:** optic tract to occipital cortex, lesion at any point (e.g. vascular, tumour) Note: Incomplete lesion results in macular (central) vision sparing	
7	**Upper quadrant homonymous hemianopia:** temporal lobe lesion (e.g. vascular, tumour)	
8	**Lower quadrant homonymous hemianopia:** parietal lobe lesion	

(b)

Figure 7.4 **(a)** Testing the visual fields by confrontation. Compare your visual fields with those of the patient (both eyes, then cover one eye) and watch the patient to ensure the patient's eye is staring directly ahead. (Courtesy of Glenn McCulloch). **(b)** Visual field defects associated with lesions of the visual system.

The third (oculomotor), fourth (trochlear) and sixth (abducens) nerves

These nerves control eye movements, the upper eyelid and pupil size, and are usually tested together.

1. Look at the pupils, noting the shape, relative sizes and any associated ptosis (complete or partial involuntary eyelid closure).
   - If one pupil, or both pupils, is small this is called **miosis**. Causes include eye drops for glaucoma, narcotics, Horner's syndrome (interruption of the sympathetic innervation of the eye, which also causes ptosis of the eyelid), a pontine brain haemorrhage and, rarely, syphilis—the Argyll Robertson pupil.
   - Enlargement of the pupils is called **mydriasis**. Causes include a third nerve palsy (unilateral), instillation of mydriatic eye drops, Adie's pupil (a ciliary ganglion lesion), trauma and iritis with synechiae.
   - Unequal pupils may be physiological and this condition is called **essential anisocoria**.
2. Use a pocket torch, shining the light from the side to gauge the **reaction** of the pupils to light. Assess quickly both the normal **direct** (constriction of the illuminated pupil) and normal **consensual** (constriction of the other pupil) responses. Remember that *both* pupils should normally contract briskly and equally when a light is shone into one.
3. Test **accommodation** (the constriction of the pupils that occurs when the eyes focus on a near object) by asking the patient to look into the distance and then at an object (e.g. a hatpin or a pen) placed about 20 cm from the nose.
4. Assess **eye movements** with both eyes first, getting the patient to follow the pin or your finger laterally right and left, then up and down (in an H pattern). Look for failure of movement.

T&O'C examination hint box

Remember that the lateral rectus muscle, supplied by the sixth nerve, only moves the eye horizontally outwards—see Figure 8.2.

---

5. Ask about **diplopia** (double vision) and in which direction of gaze the diplopia is most pronounced. Diplopia may be

due to weakness of one or more of the ocular muscles. The separation of the images is greatest in the direction in which the affected muscle has its dominant effect.

6. Look for **nystagmus**. This is an involuntary rhythmic oscillation of the ocular muscles back and forth. It may be:
   - **pendular**, where the oscillations of the eye occur centrally and are equal in each direction—this usually indicates a problem with fixation
   - **phasic** (jerky), which involves a slow drifting movement and a rapid correcting movement.

The direction of the nystagmus is defined as the direction of the fast phase. Phasic nystagmus is a sign of cerebellar, brainstem or vestibular disease. Fine phasic nystagmus is normal at the extremes of gaze, so testing should involve asking the patient to follow your finger so that each eye is abducted about 30° in turn.

T&O'C examination hint box

Remember the characteristic signs of palsies of the third, fourth and fifth nerves:
- *third nerve:* ipsilateral (same side as the lesion) mydriasis that is unreactive to light or accommodation, complete ptosis and divergent strabismus (the eye is deviated down and out)
- *fourth nerve:* inability to turn the eye down and in; the patient's head may be tilted away from the abnormal side
- *sixth nerve:* failure of lateral movement, with diplopia most pronounced on looking laterally on the affected side.

The fifth (trigeminal) nerve

1. Test the **corneal reflexes** gently using a wisp of cottonwool to touch the cornea and ask the patient whether the touch can be felt. Normally *both* the eyelids should shut briskly. The sensory component of this reflex is the fifth nerve and the motor component is the seventh nerve.

2. Test **facial sensation** in the three divisions: ophthalmic, maxillary and mandibular (see Fig 7.5).

3. Test **pain** (pin-prick) **sensation** with a new disposable neurology pin in each area. Start on one side of the forehead and move to the other side, pressing the pin into the skin and asking the patient to tell you what he or she

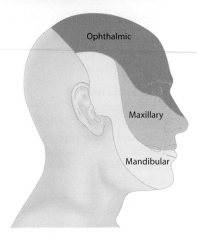

Figure 7.5   The divisions of the trigeminal nerve.

feels (sharp is normal!). If areas of reduced sensation (dull) are found, map them by moving the pin until normal sensation is again present (sharp).

4. Test **light touch** by touching but not stroking the skin with a piece of cottonwool.

5. Note the presence of **sensory dissociation** (usually loss of pain and temperature sensation and preservation of light touch). This is rare but occurs typically in syringobulbia, where enlargement of the central canal of the brainstem and upper spinal cord interrupts crossing pain and temperature fibres first.

6. Examine the **motor** division of the fifth nerve by asking the patient to **clench** the teeth while you feel the masseter muscles. Then to **open** his or her mouth while you attempt to **force it closed** (not too hard); this should not be possible if the pterygoid muscles are working. A unilateral lesion causes the jaw to deviate towards the weak (affected) side because the normal muscle's action is unopposed.

7. Test the **jaw jerk** by tapping the reflex hammer on your own thumb placed on the chin of the patient, whose mouth is partly open. This is present in healthy people, but is exaggerated, with brisk bilateral contraction of the masseter

muscles, in cases of pseudobulbar palsy (bilateral upper motor neuron lesions also affecting the ninth, tenth and twelfth nerves).

The seventh (facial) nerve

Test the muscles of **facial expression**.

1. Ask the patient to look up and *wrinkle the forehead*. Look for loss of wrinkling and feel the muscle strength by pushing down on each side. This is preserved in an upper motor neuron lesion because of bilateral cortical representation of these muscles.

2. Next ask the patient to *shut his or her eyes tightly* and compare the two sides. Both upper and lower unilateral facial weakness can lead to incomplete closure of the eye on the same side, but a lower motor neuron lesion has a more pronounced effect.

3. Finally, ask the patient to *grin* and compare the nasolabial grooves. The side on which the groove is less pronounced (flatter) is the abnormal one.

The eighth (acoustic) nerve

Quantitative hearing assessment is not possible without special equipment, but useful qualitative information can be obtained at the bedside.

1. Whisper a number 60 cm away from each of the patient's ears while the other ear is distracted by movement of your finger near the auditory canal. It takes practice to know at what level of loudness a whisper is normally audible.

2. If there is deafness, perform **Rinne's** and **Weber's** tests and examine the external auditory canals and the eardrums (see Ch 8).

The ninth (glossopharyngeal) and tenth (vagus) nerves

1. Look at the palate and note any **uvular displacement**. Ask the patient to say 'ah' and look for symmetrical movement of the soft palate. With a unilateral lesion of the tenth nerve the uvula is drawn towards the unaffected (normal) side.

2. It may be unwise to test even gently for a **gag reflex** (the **ninth** nerve is the sensory component and the **tenth** nerve the motor component), whereby a spatula is touched onto

each side of the soft palate in turn. The normal response is gagging with contraction of the palate on both sides, or even vomiting.

3. To test the sensory (afferent) limb of the gag reflex, it is preferable to **touch the pharynx on each side**, and ask whether the touch can be felt and seems the same on each side. The motor (efferent) limb of this reflex would have been tested when the patient said 'aah'.

4. Ask the patient to speak to assess **hoarseness**, and to cough and to swallow. A 'bovine' or hollow cough suggests bilateral recurrent laryngeal nerve lesions.

The eleventh (accessory) nerve

1. Ask the patient to shrug his or her shoulders and feel the **trapezius** as you push the shoulders down.

2. Then ask the patient to turn his or her head against resistance and feel the bulk of the **sternocleidomastoid**. The left sternocleidomastoid turns the head to the right, and vice versa. Nerve palsy (a lower motor neuron lesion) causes weak contraction of the sternocleidomastoid muscle ipsilateral to the lesion (i.e. weakness of head turning to the opposite side). An upper motor neuron lesion may cause weakness of contralateral head version because of ipsilateral sternomastoid weakness.

The twelfth (hypoglossal) nerve

1. While examining the mouth, inspect the **tongue** for **wasting** and **fasciculation** (random flickering movements of small muscle groups), which is characteristic of a lower motor neuron lesion.

T&O'C examination hint box

The presence of fasciculations of the tongue is an important sign and easily missed. Ask the patient to rest the tongue on the floor of the mouth. You need to be patient to allow time for fasciculations to appear.

2. Next ask the patient to **protrude the tongue**. A unilateral lesion causes the tongue to deviate towards the weaker (affected) side.

T&O'C examination essentials

Upper versus lower motor neuron lesions
Remember the difference between upper and lower motor neuron lesions (see Figs 7.6 and 7.7).

- A lesion that interrupts the neural pathway above the anterior horn cell in the spinal cord is called an **upper motor neuron lesion**. Examples include lesions of the cortex, internal capsule, brainstem and spinal cord. These are associated with increased tone (spasticity) in the affected muscle groups. The reflexes are exaggerated and clonus (a rhythmical muscle contraction) may be present, but muscle wasting and fasciculations are absent.
- **Lower motor neuron lesions** result in reduced tone and reflexes, muscle wasting and sometimes fasciculations.

Signs of upper motor neuron lesions
1. Weakness is present in all muscle groups of the lower limb but may be more marked in the flexor muscles. In the upper limb, weakness may be more marked in the extensors (pattern-extended leg, flexed arm). There is very little muscle wasting (unless from disuse).
2. Increased tone is present (may be clasp-knife—initial resistance that gives way suddenly) and is often associated with clonus.
3. The reflexes are increased except for the superficial reflexes (e.g. abdominal), which are absent.
4. There is an extensor (Babinski) plantar response (upgoing toe).

Signs of lower motor neuron lesions
1. Weakness may be more obvious distally than proximally, and the flexor and extensor muscles are equally involved. Wasting is a prominent feature.
2. Tone is reduced.
3. The reflexes are reduced and the plantar response is normal or absent.
4. Fasciculations may be present.

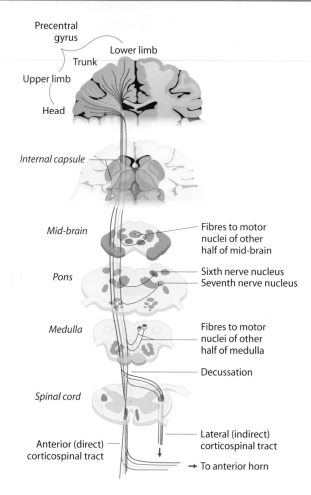

Figure 7.6 Motor pathways.

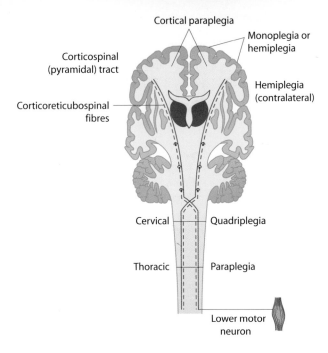

Cortical paraplegia

Monoplegia or
hemiplegia

Corticospinal
(pyramidal) tract

Hemiplegia
(contralateral)

Corticoreticubospinal
fibres

Cervical | Quadriplegia

Thoracic | Paraplegia

Lower motor
neuron

Figure 7.7 Upper and lower motor neuron lesions.

UPPER LIMBS

Ask the patient to sit over the side of the bed facing you. Look
for abnormal movements.

1. A **tremor** is rhythmical oscillation around a joint due to
   contraction and relaxation of muscles or alternating
   contraction and relaxation in opposing muscle groups. A
   normal, fine (>10 cycles/second) tremor is present when
   muscles attempt to maintain a stationary position against
   gravity (**physiological tremor**). This is exaggerated with
   anxiety, alcoholism and thyrotoxicosis, and in patients
   with a familial tremor. A coarse **resting tremor** occurs
   in Parkinson's disease: there is repetitive flexion and
   contraction of the fingers, and abduction and adduction of
   the thumb (pill-rolling tremor) at rest. An **intention
   tremor** becomes more pronounced as the limb is directed

towards an object—for example, if the patient reaches out to touch something.

2. **Irregular movements.**
   - **Choreiform** movements are involuntary jerky repetitive movements that may appear to be semi-purposeful; they occur in extrapyramidal disease. Flapping of the tongue (rapid protrusion and retraction with flapping of the tip) is commonly associated.
   - **Athetosis** is a slow, writhing movement.
   - **Myoclonic jerks** are involuntary sudden shock-like muscle contractions that are relatively common.
   - **Hemiballismus**, characterised by dramatic involuntary swinging movements, is rare.
3. **Pseudoathetosis** (small writhing movements, especially of the fingers) occurs because of proprioceptive (posterior column) loss.

Motor system

Examine the motor system systematically every time.

1. Inspect first for **wasting** (both proximal and distal) and **fasciculations**. Don't forget to include the trunk and shoulder girdle in your inspection.
2. Ask the patient to hold out both hands with the arms extended and to close the eyes. Look for **drifting of one or both arms**, which can be due to (1) upper motor neuron weakness, (2) a cerebellar lesion or (3) proprioceptive loss.
3. Feel the **muscle bulk** of the upper arms and forearms and note any muscle tenderness.
4. Test **tone** at the wrists and elbows by moving the joints passively at varying velocities. Flex and extend the patient's wrists and elbows after asking him or her to relax and not help you. It takes some practice to become familiar with normal muscle tone.[3] Changes in tone are easier to detect if they are unilateral.
5. Assess **power** (see Fig 7.8) at the shoulders, elbows, wrists and fingers. Remember that right-handed people are

---

3 There is no resistance to these passive movements in young cooperative patients and therefore they cannot really have reduced tone.

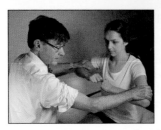

'Stop me pushing your arms down'

(a) Shoulder abduction

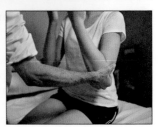

'Stop me pulling your arms up'

(b) Shoulder adduction

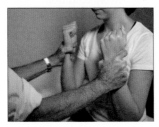

'Stop me straightening your elbow'

(c) Elbow flexion

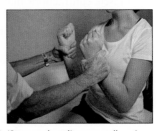

'Stop me bending your elbow'

(d) Elbow extension

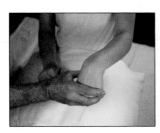

'Stop me straightening your hand'

(e) Wrist flexion

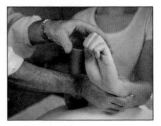

'Stop me bending your wrist down'

(f) Wrist extension

Figure 7.8 Testing power in the upper limbs.

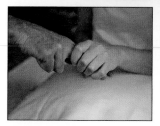

'Squeeze my fingers hard'

(g) Finger flexion

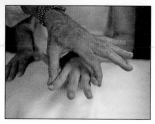

'Stop me bringing your fingers together'
(h) Finger abduction

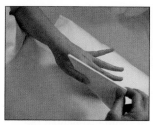

'Hold the paper and stop me pulling it out'
(i) Froment's sign

Figure 7.8, continued

slightly stronger on the right side. Power is graded as follows:[4]

0: complete paralysis
1: a flicker of contraction
2: movement is possible where gravity is excluded
3: movement is possible against gravity but not if any further resistance is added
4: movement is possible against gravity and some resistance
5: normal power.

---

4 Remember that your own strength may be different from the patient's. It is sometimes alarming to see a powerful medical student testing power in a frail elderly person.

Shoulder

- **Abduction** (C5, C6 nerve root innervation): the patient should abduct the arms with the elbows flexed and resist your attempt to push them down (see Fig 7.8a).
- **Adduction** (C6, C7, C8): the patient should adduct the arms with the elbows flexed and not allow you to separate them (see Fig 7.8b).

Elbow

- **Flexion** (C5, C6): the patient should bend the elbow and pull so as not to let you straighten it out (see Fig 7.8c).
- **Extension** (C7): the patient should bend the elbow and push so as not to let you bend it (see Fig 7.8d).

Wrist

- **Flexion** (C6, C7, C8): the patient should bend the wrist and not allow you to straighten it (see Fig 7.8e).
- **Extension** (C7, C8): the patient should extend the wrist and not allow you to bend it (see Fig 7.8f).

Fingers

- **Extension** (C7, C8): the patient should straighten the fingers and not allow you to push them down (push with the side of your hand across the patient's metacarpophalangeal joints).
- **Flexion** (C7, C8): the patient squeezes two of your fingers (see Fig 7.8g).
- **Abduction** (C8, T1): the patient should spread out the fingers and not allow you to push them together (see Fig 7.8h).
- Look for **wasting of the small muscles of the hand** with deep gutters between the long extensor tendons and hypothenar eminence (ulnar nerve lesion) or thenar eminence (median nerve lesion). Ask the patient to extend both wrists and ask about tingling (**Phalen's sign** from median nerve entrapment in the carpal tunnel syndrome).
- If the patient has a **claw hand** (fixed flexion of the fingers), testing for an **ulnar** or a **median** nerve lesion is necessary.
- When the patient grasps a piece of paper between the thumb and the lateral aspect of the forefinger, the thumb flexes if an ulnar lesion has caused loss of the adductor of the thumb (**Froment's sign**; see Fig 7.8i).

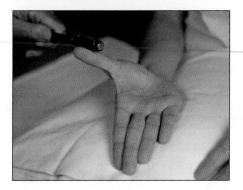

Figure 7.9 The pen-touching test for loss of abductor pollicis brevis (median nerve). 'Lift your thumb to touch my pen, but keep your hand flat on the table.'

- Ask the patient to place his or her hand flat, with the palm upwards, and then ask the patient to lift the thumb vertically against resistance or to lift the thumb vertically to touch your pen (**pen-touching test** for loss of abductor pollicis brevis—median nerve; see Fig 7.9). This is not possible if there is a median nerve palsy at the wrist or above.

Reflexes

Examine the reflexes (see Fig 7.10) routinely at the elbow and wrist. Remember that the **reflex arc** consists of afferent (sensory) and efferent (motor) pathways. The afferent pathway is stimulated when a tendon is stretched (e.g. after being struck by a reflex hammer). This pathway synapses in the spinal cord with a motor neuron that fires, stimulating the efferent pathway, and causes contraction of the attached muscle to release the stretch on the tendon. Interruption of the efferent or afferent limb of the reflex arc prevents contraction and the reflex is absent. Interruption of pathways in the spinal cord above the level of the motor neuron (upper motor neuron lesion) releases this from inhibition and causes exaggerated reflexes. Reflexes may be normal, increased (upper motor neuron lesion), decreased or even absent (lower motor neuron lesion)

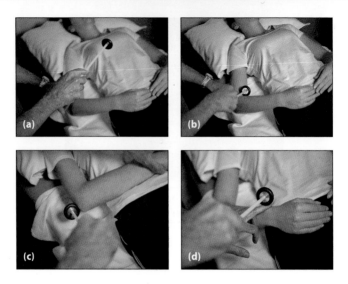

Figure 7.10 The biceps **(a and b)** and triceps **(c)** jerks and brachioradialis **(d)**.

or delayed (contraction is brisk but return is slow—typical of hypothyroidism).[5]

Clonus is rhythmical contraction of the muscle that can continue as long as tension is maintained on the tendon. This occurs with an upper motor neuron lesion. Clonus is not usually tested in the upper limbs.

An idea of the range of normal reflexes can only be obtained by practice. Upper limb tendon reflexes are sometimes difficult to elicit in younger patients.

T&O'C examination hint box

Patients have left and right sides for a purpose (i.e. to allow medical students to compare one side with the other). The normal symmetry of neurological findings is your friend. Even very striking asymmetry will be missed by the student who does not compare one side with the other.

---

5 Attempts to grade reflexes on a more complicated scale than this is of minimal value.

- **Biceps** (C5, C6): place your left forefinger over the biceps tendon and allow the patellar hammer to fall onto it (see Fig 7.10a,b). There is normally a brisk (but not too brisk) contraction of the biceps muscle.
- **Triceps** (C7, C8): support one of the patient's elbows with one hand and tap over the triceps tendon with the hammer (see Fig 7.10c). There is normally triceps contraction and extension of the forearm.
- **Brachioradialis** (C5, C6): place a few of your fingers over the distal end of the radius and strike them (see Fig 7.10d). Contraction of the brachioradialis causes flexion of the elbow.
- **Finger** (C8, T1): interlock your hand with the patient's while the patient's hand is resting palm upwards and use the tendon hammer to strike your hand. Normally, there is slight flexion of all fingers and of the interphalangeal joint of the thumb.
- In patients with suspected upper motor neuron disease, look for **Hoffman's reflex**: the terminal part of the patient's middle finger is flicked downwards between your thumb and finger; it is abnormal if the thumb flexes and adducts while the other fingers flex. The presence of this reflex indicates hyper-reflexia but is not pathognomonic of an upper motor neuron disease.

T&O'C examination essentials

Remember that motor weakness can be due to:
- an **upper motor neuron lesion** (hyper-reflexia with absence of wasting)
- a **lower motor neuron lesion** (wasting due to denervation, absent reflexes)
- **neuromuscular transmission disorders** (fatigue on repeated muscle use)
- a **myopathy** (muscle disease usually with wasting but with variable reflexes).

If there is evidence of a lower motor neuron lesion, consider anterior horn cell, nerve root or brachial plexus lesions, peripheral nerve lesions or a motor peripheral neuropathy.

Coordination (cerebellar function)

1. First apply **finger–nose** testing. Ask the patient to touch the tip of your forefinger (the target) with his or her own

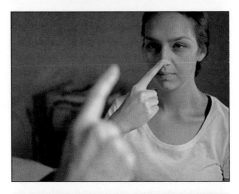

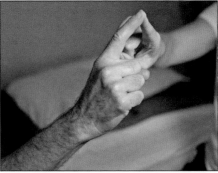

Figure 7.11 The cerebellar examination: finger–nose test. 'Touch your nose and then my finger.'

forefinger and with the arm extended, and then to touch his or her own nose (see Fig 7.11). Alternate the movements rapidly. Cerebellar disease will cause the patient's finger to oscillate and overshoot.

2. Examine for **dysdiadochokinesis**, an inability to perform rapidly alternating movements, such as supinating and pronating the wrists repeatedly (this action appears clumsy in the presence of cerebellar disease).

3. Next look for **rebound**. Ask the patient to lift both arms quickly from his or her sides then stop halfway. Rebound is present if the patient cannot stop one or both arms.

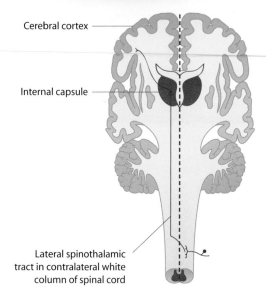

Figure 7.12 Pain and temperature pathways.

SENSORY SYSTEM

Examine the sensory system after motor testing because this can be time-consuming.

1. First test the **spinothalamic pathway** (**pain** and **temperature**; see Fig 7.12). Demonstrate to the patient the sharpness of a new disposable neurology pin,[6] then ask the patient to close his or her eyes and tell you whether the sensation is sharp or dull. Start proximally and test pin-prick sensation in each dermatome (see Fig 7.13). As you are assessing, try to determine whether any sensory loss is:

   - **dermatomal** (loss fits into the pattern of one or more dermatomes—cord or nerve root lesion)

---

6 The traditional testing of the sensation of sharpness on the upper sternum causes distress (and annoyance) to oncologists who see patients with malignancy in the upper thoracic spine and therefore abnormal sensation on the upper chest wall.

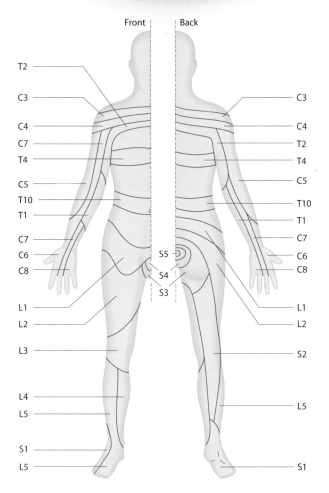

Figure 7.13 The dermatomes of the limbs and trunk.

- **peripheral nerve** (pattern specific for the nerve affected, e.g. median or ulnar nerve; see Fig 7.14)
- **peripheral neuropathy** (affected area is in the shape of a glove)
- **hemisensory** (loss involves one side—cortical or cord pattern of loss).

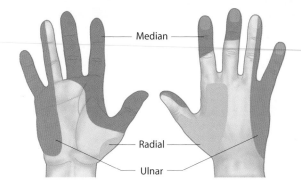

Median

Radial

Ulnar

Figure 7.14   Sensory loss of the median and ulnar nerves on the hand.

Always compare each side and, as you move up the arms, note the presence of a sensory level (the level of change from abnormal to normal). Tap the pin a number of times in each place to ensure reproducibility.

2. Next test the **posterior column pathway** (**vibration** and **proprioception**; see Fig 7.15).

- Use a 128-Hz tuning fork to assess vibration sense. Place the vibrating fork on a distal interphalangeal joint when the patient has his or her eyes closed and ask whether the vibrations can be felt. If so, ask the patient to tell you when the vibration ceases and then, after a short wait, stop the fork vibrating. If the patient has deficient sensation, test at the wrist, then the elbow and then at the shoulder to determine the level of the sensory loss.

- Examine proprioception first with the distal interphalangeal joint of the index finger. When the patient has his or her eyes open, grasp the distal phalanx from the sides and move it up and down to demonstrate. Then ask the patient to close his or her eyes and repeat the manoeuvre, and stop with the phalanx in the up or down position. Repeat this a few times, ending with the phalanx in a different position each time. Normally, movement through even a few degrees is detectable, and the patient can tell whether it is up or down. If there is an abnormality, proceed to test the wrist and elbows similarly to determine the level of the lesion.

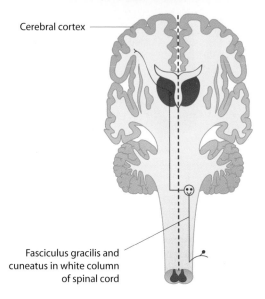

Cerebral cortex

Fasciculus gracilis and
cuneatus in white column
of spinal cord

Figure 7.15 Vibration and joint position sense pathways.

3. Test **light touch** with cottonwool. Touch the skin lightly in each dermatome. Do not wipe the skin as tickle is a spinothalamic sensation and the ticklish patient may be unable to keep still.

4. Test for **cortical sensory abnormalities** if a cortical lesion is suspected after the initial examination. Parietal lobe lesions may cause **sensory inattention**. Here, sensation is normal when one side at a time is tested, but absent on the opposite side to the lesion if both sides are tested together. The patient shuts his or her eyes and both hands are touched. The stimulus is felt only on the normal side. **Astereognosis** also occurs with parietal lesions. This refers

to a patient's inability to recognise an object placed in his or her hand.

LOWER LIMBS

Gait

Difficulty with walking is a common problem. First consider the range of possible causes, then ask about the problem (see Questions box 7.1). Finally, test the stance and gait, if possible (see Fig 7.16).

T&O'C examination hint box

If you are told in an exam that a patient has difficulty walking, start by asking the patient to walk.

Questions box 7.1 Questions to ask the patient who has difficulty with walking

! denotes a possible urgent or dangerous problem

1. How long have you had difficulty walking? Can you walk at all?
2. Is it getting worse?
3. Did it begin suddenly? (CVA, acute spinal problem—injury, sepsis, thrombosis)
4. Have you been generally unwell or had a fever?
5. Is one leg weak? (Most often CVA)
6. Have you injured your leg or back?
! 7. Have you had difficulty passing urine or moving your bowels? (Spinal cord lesion)
8. Is there a problem with your balance? (Cerebellar disease, peripheral neuropathy, Parkinson's disease)
9. Have you had problems with tremors or shakes?
! 10. Have you had any falls as a result of the problem with your walking?
11. Have you needed to use a walking stick or a frame?
12. Have you had arthritis, gout or pain in your joints or feet?
13. Do you have difficulty getting up from a chair? (Proximal myopathy)
14. Are you taking any medications such as cortisone or prednisone? (Proximal myopathy)
15. Are you diabetic? If so, for how long have you been diabetic?
16. Have you had cancer? (Spinal metastases)
17. Are you limited by pain in the calves when you walk a certain distance? (Claudication)

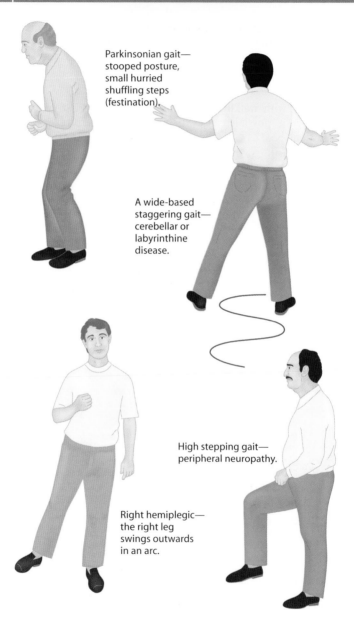

Parkinsonian gait—stooped posture, small hurried shuffling steps (festination).

A wide-based staggering gait—cerebellar or labyrinthine disease.

High stepping gait—peripheral neuropathy.

Right hemiplegic—the right leg swings outwards in an arc.

Figure 7.16 Gait disturbances.

1. Ask the patient to walk normally for a short distance and then to turn around quickly and come back. Then ask the patient to walk heel-to-toe, placing one foot just in front of the other (a test of cerebellar function that has been used by the police to test for alcohol intoxication in less sophisticated times). Next ask the patient to walk on the toes (difficult or impossible with an S1 or tibial nerve lesion). Finally ask the patient to walk on the heels (difficult or impossible with an L4–5 or peroneal nerve lesion).

2. Ask the patient to stand with his or her feet together, first with the eyes open and then with them closed. Increased swaying when the eyes are open suggests cerebellar disease. If this occurs only when the eyes are closed (**Romberg's sign**), it suggests proprioceptive loss.

T&O'C examination essentials: Difficulty walking

Important differential diagnoses
- Neurological disease
    - Upper motor neuron weakness
    - Lower motor neuron weakness
    - Motor neuron disease
    - Myasthenia gravis
    - Cerebellar disorder
    - Movement disorder
    - Peripheral neuropathy
    - Myopathy
- Hysteria
- Musculoskeletal disease
    - Injury
    - Arthritis
- Peripheral vascular disease

T&O'C examination hint box

Gait examinations are common in OSCE exams. You will be expected to have an understanding of Romberg's test and the meaning of a positive Romberg's sign (increased swaying with eyes closed). Practise this test and learn how to avoid having patients fall over when they close their eyes.

Motor system

1. Lay the patient in bed with the legs entirely exposed. Place a towel over the groin—note whether a urinary catheter is present.
2. Look for **muscle wasting** and **fasciculations**. Note any tremor.
3. Feel the **muscle bulk** of the **quadriceps** and then run your hand up each shin, feeling for wasting of the **anterior tibial** muscles.
4. Test **tone** at the knees and ankles. Ask the patient to relax and not to oppose or assist your movement of the limbs. Place your hand under the patient's knee and lift the knee quickly so that it flexes and extends. Then grasp the foot and flex and extend it repeatedly. With practice, normal and abnormal muscle resistance to these movements will be appreciated.
5. Test **clonus**. Push the lower end of the quadriceps sharply down towards the knee. Sustained rhythmical contractions of the quadriceps indicate an upper motor neuron lesion. Also test the ankle by sharply dorsiflexing the foot with the knee bent and the thigh externally rotated; look for clonus of the calf muscles.
6. Assess **power** next at the hips, knees and ankles (see Fig 7.17). This should again be graded from 0 to 5 (see p. 206).

Hip

- **Flexion** (L2, L3 innervation): ask the patient to lift up the straight leg and not to let you push it down (having placed your hand above the knee; see Fig 7.17a).
- **Extension** (S1): ask the patient to keep the leg down and not to let you pull it up from underneath the calf or ankle (see Fig 7.17b).
- **Abduction** (L5): ask the patient to abduct the leg and not to let you push it in.
- **Adduction** (L2, L3): ask the patient to keep the leg adducted and not to let you push it out.

Knee

- **Flexion** (L5, S1): ask the patient to bend the knee and not to let you straighten it (see Fig 7.17c).
- **Extension** (L3, L4): with the knee slightly bent, ask the patient to straighten the knee and not to let you bend it (see Fig 7.17d).

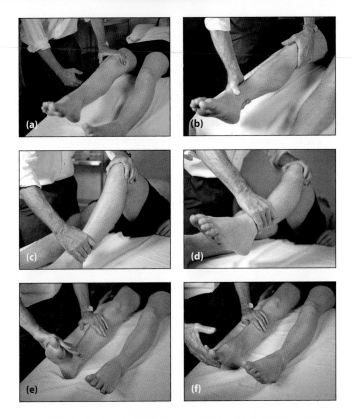

Figure 7.17   Testing power in the lower limbs. **(a)** 'Lift your leg up against my hand' (hip flexion). **(b)** 'Stop me lifting your leg' (hip extension). **(c)** 'Bend your heel up towards your bottom' (knee flexion). **(d)** 'Try to straighten your leg against my hand' (knee extension). **(e)** 'Bend your foot up towards your knee against my hand' (plantar (ankle) flexion). **(f)** 'Push your foot down against my hand' (dorsiflexion— extension of the ankle).

Ankle

- **Plantarflexion** (S1, S2): ask the patient to push the foot down and not to let you push it up (see Fig 7.17e).
- **Dorsiflexion** (L4, L5): ask the patient to bring the foot up and not to let you push it down (see Fig 7.17f).
- **Eversion** (L5): ask the patient to evert the foot against resistance.
- **Inversion** (L5, S1): with the foot in complete plantarflexion, ask the patient to invert the foot against resistance.

Reflexes

Examine the **reflexes** (see Fig 7.18).

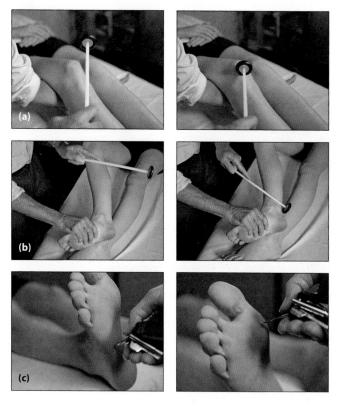

Figure 7.18 **(a)** Knee jerk. **(b)** Ankle jerk. **(c)** Plantar reflexes.

Knee (L3, L4)
- Allow the patellar hammer to fall elegantly onto the infrapatellar tendon while the patient's knee is supported by your arm (see Fig 7.18a). Watch for contraction of the quadriceps.

Ankle (S1, S2)
- The patient's foot is in the mid-position at the ankle, the knee is bent and the thigh is externally rotated on the bed. Allow the patellar hammer to fall onto the Achilles tendon (see Fig 7.18b). Plantar flexion of the foot will normally occur.
- The reflex can also be elicited by having the patient kneel and directly tapping the tendon.

Plantar response (L5, S1, S2)
- Run an expensive motor car key or similar object slowly along the lateral aspect of the patient's sole (see Fig 7.18c). The normal response is flexion of the great toe. Upper motor neuron lesions result in extension (dorsiflexion) of the great toe and fanning of the other toes. This is described as an upgoing (extensor) plantar response or a **Babinski sign**. This sign is normal in infants.

T&O'C examination hint box

The plantar response can be uncomfortable for the patient. Warn the patient what you are about to do and do not scrape too hard. Practise on willing colleagues until you find out how much pressure is tolerable and how sharp the key should be.

Coordination (cerebellar function)

1. Perform the **heel–shin** test. Ask the patient to run the heel of one foot up and down the shin of the other leg as rapidly and accurately as possible. Look for wobbling or the heel falling off (see Fig 7.19).
2. Perform the **toe–finger** test. Ask the patient to bring the toe up to touch your forefinger with the knee bent (see Fig 7.20). Look for tremor and overshooting.
3. Perform **tapping of the feet**. Ask the patient to tap the sole of the foot on your hand. Look for clumsy or slow movements (**dysdiadochokinesis**).

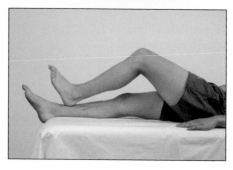

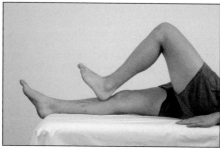

Figure 7.19 Test coordination: heel–shin test. 'Lift your right leg up, place your heel on your left knee and then run it quickly down your shin.' (Courtesy of Glenn McCulloch.)

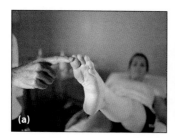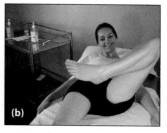

Figure 7.20 **(a)** The toe–finger test. **(b)** And a patient attempting the toe–nose test (toe–nose testing is not part of the examination and is included for amusement only).

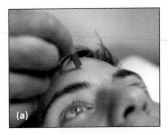 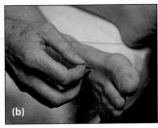

Figure 7.21 **(a)** Demonstrating sharpness on the forehead. **(b)** 'Shut your eyes. Tell me when I touch you, does that feel sharp? Is it the same as on the other side?'

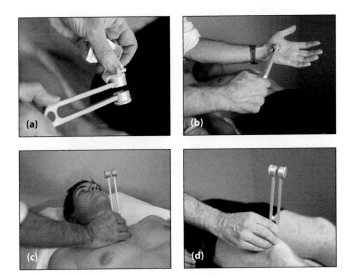

Figure 7.22 **(a)** 128-Hz tuning fork. **(b)** Tap fork. **(c)** Demonstrate vibration on the sternum. **(d)** 'Shut your eyes. Can you feel that vibrating? Tell me when it stops.'

Sensory system

1. Test **pain** (pin-prick; see Fig 7.21), then **vibration** (see Fig 7.22) and **proprioception** (see Fig 7.23), and then **light touch** (as described for the upper limbs and in each dermatome on both sides; see Fig 7.13). If sensory loss

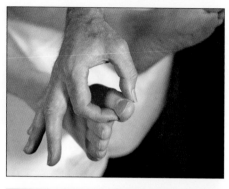

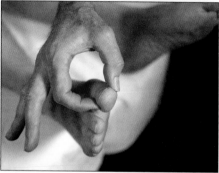

Figure 7.23 Testing proprioception of the toe. 'Shut your eyes and tell me whether I have moved your toe up or down.'

involves the entire leg or both legs, attempt to establish where normal sensation begins on the trunk or chest (the sensory level).

2. Test the **abdominal reflexes** (see Fig 7.24). Stroke the skin of the lower abdominal wall in each quadrant with a sharpish object such as a key or wooden spatula (not the one previously used to test the gag reflex), first on one side and then on the other. Brisk contraction of the underlying muscles normally occurs. Test the upper and lower quadrants on both sides. Absent reflexes may be a result of an upper motor neuron lesion, but lax abdominal muscles or previous surgery that has cut the superficial abdominal nerves may also cause loss of this reflex.

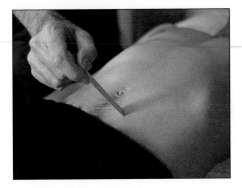

Figure 7.24 Testing the abdominal reflex.

3. Examine sensation in the **saddle region** (perineum and medial aspects of the upper thighs) region.
4. Test the **anal reflex** (S2, S3, S4); there is normally contraction of the external sphincter in response to scratching of the perianal skin.

THE SPINE

1. Examine the **back**. Look for deformity, scars and neurofibromas. Palpate for tenderness over the vertebral bodies and auscultate for bruits. Any of these may indicate spinal cord abnormalities.

> **T&O'C examination hint box**
>
> Always look for the presence of a urinary catheter: it may indicate spinal cord disease that has caused urinary retention.

2. Perform the **straight leg raising test**. Lay the patient flat and slowly flex the hip while keeping the knee fully extended. Tell the patient to advise you as soon as there is pain and where it occurs (a disc compression of the lumbar or sacral roots will limit leg raising, because of pain in the ipsilateral leg that will be increased by foot dorsiflexion). With more severe nerve root irritation the pain will be felt in the other lower limb as well (crossed straight leg raising

sign). Test the upper lumbar roots by laying the patient prone and extending the hip (while the knee is flexed to 90°) (see **femoral nerve stretch test**, p. 277).

The neurological history and examination OSCE: hints panel

1. This man has had problems with confusion. Please examine him. (Wash your hands)
   (a) General inspection:* stand back and look for signs of dehydration, malnutrition, cyanosis or recent evidence of trauma.
   (b) Test orientation for time, place and person.
   (c) Measure his pulse and blood pressure (hypertensive encephalopathy). Look for signs of cardiac failure.
   (d) Look for signs of alcoholism and liver failure.
   (e) Take his temperature and look for any obvious focus of infection.
   (f) Ask to test his urine and blood sugar (hypoglycaemia or diabetes mellitus).
   (g) Ask to review his medication chart.
   (h) Synthesise and present your findings.
2. This man has felt unsteady and clumsy. Please examine his coordination.
   (Wash your hands)
   You are considering cerebellar disease, based on the introduction.
   (a) Examine for nystagmus (typically jerky, with an increased amplitude on looking to the side of a cerebellar lesion).
   (b) Test for dysarthria (e.g. say 'British constitution'). Note any jerky, loud explosive cerebellar-type speech.
   (c) Test arm drift (hypotonia, in cerebellar disease on the same side as the lesion).
   (d) Assess the finger–nose test (for intention tremor and past pointing) and rapidly alternating movements (dysdiadokinesis). Then test rebound.
   (e) Assess leg tone, then the heel–skin test, intention tremor (big toe to your finger) and heel tapping on the other shin.
   (f) Ask the patient to fold his arms and sit up (truncal ataxia).
   (g) Assess gait (staggering towards the side of the cerebellar lesion).
   (h) Examine the cranial nerves (e.g. fifth, seventh and eighth lesions on one side from a cerebellopontine angle tumour).
   (i) Auscultate over the skull for a cerebellar bruit.
   (j) Auscultate for carotid bruits.
   (k) Synthesise and present your findings.

---

* Delirium or confusion is usually a multifactorial condition.

3. This woman has had trouble walking. Please examine her. (Wash your hands)

(a) Undress the patient to the underpants.

(b) Make a general inspection for:
- wasting or asymmetry of the lower limbs—peripheral wasting and pes cavus suggests an inherited ataxia (e.g. Friederich's ataxia); wasting of one side suggests a lower motor neuron problem with the spine, nerve roots or peripheral nerve
- joint deformity, swelling or erythema
- the presence of a urinary catheter
- abnormal movements (e.g. Parkinsonian tremor).

(c) Ask the patient to walk—if necessary with a frame or stick but preferably just with your help. Note:
- any difficulty getting up from the chair
- hemiplegic gait
- wide-based (ataxic) gait (cerebellar disease, peripheral neuropathy).

(d) If the patient manages to walk, ask her to:
- turn and walk back
- walk heel-to-toe
- perform Romberg's test
- stand on her heels and then on her toes (tests L5/S1)
- squat and stand (tests proximal muscle strength).

(e) Ask the patient to lie down.
- Make a careful inspection for wasting and fasciculations.
- Look for joint abnormalities.
- Test tone.
- Test power.
- Test the reflexes, including the Babinski sign.
- Test cerebellar function.
- Test position and vibration sense.
- Test pain sensation.
- Feel for the peripheral pulses, if indicated from the history.

(f) Look at the spine for scars and tenderness.

(g) Consider a diagnosis and the differential diagnosis.

T&O'C examination essentials

The neurological examination

1. A careful neurological history should direct the neurological examination to the most relevant areas. Symptoms may occur before signs can be detected, but in the absence of symptoms any signs are less likely to be important.
2. The methodical approach that characterises the skilled neurological examination helps define the anatomical site of the abnormality.
3. A careful neurological examination will usually enable you to develop a sensible differential diagnosis.
4. Note the distribution of signs and look particularly for asymmetrical abnormalities.
5. Healthy people may have no gag or abdominal reflexes.
6. Absent tendon reflexes usually indicate an abnormality in the sensory or motor system.
7. An extensor plantar reflex that is reproducible is never normal (except in infants).
8. Hepatitis B and C virus, and HIV, have been isolated from needles used to test pin-prick sensation. Disposable needles should always be used.

The eyes, ears, nose and throat

Failure to examine the throat is a glaring sin of omission, especially in children. One finger in the throat and one in the rectum makes a good diagnostician.

Sir William Osler (1849–1919)

The examination of the eyes, ears, nose and throat is usually directed by the history. These small parts of the body may provide vital diagnostic clues in neurological or systemic disease.

The eyes

EXAMINATION ANATOMY

The structure of the eye is shown in Figure 8.1. Keep in mind the anatomy as you examine the eyes, as set out below. Figure 8.2 shows the muscles responsible for eye movements and their innervation.

EXAMINATION METHOD

1. Sit the patient at the edge of the bed facing you. Standing well back from the patient, inspect for:
   - **ptosis** (drooping of one or both upper eyelids)
   - **colour of the sclerae**:

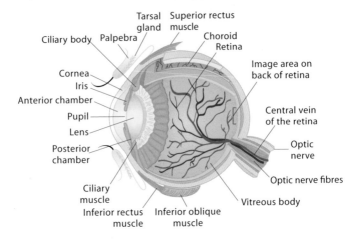

Figure 8.1 The structure of the eye.

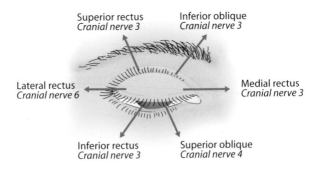

Figure 8.2 Eye movements, muscles and innervation (right eye).

- yellow (deposits of bilirubin in jaundice)
- blue (which may be due to osteogenesis imperfecta, because the thin sclerae allow the choroidal pigment to show through; blue sclerae can also occur in families without osteogenesis imperfecta)
- red (**iritis**, which causes central inflammation; **conjunctivitis**, which causes more peripheral

inflammation often with pus; or **subconjunctival haemorrhage** as a result of trauma)
- scleral pallor, which occurs in anaemia. Pull down the lower lid and look for the normal contrast between the pearly white posterior conjunctiva and the red anterior part. Loss of this contrast is a reliable sign of anaemia.

2. Look from behind and above the patient for **exophthalmos**, which is prominence of the eyes—if there is actual protrusion of the eyes from the orbits, this is called **proptosis** and is best detected by looking at the eyes from above the forehead; protrusion beyond the supraorbital ridge is abnormal. If exophthalmos is present, examine specifically for thyroid eye disease (p. 247).

3. Proceed as for the cranial nerve examination—that is, testing visual acuity, visual fields (see Fig 7.4) and pupillary responses to light and accommodation. Look for an **afferent pupillary defect** (or Marcus Gunn sign). Move the torch in an arc from pupil to pupil—an abnormal pupil will paradoxically dilate when the torch is moved to the abnormal eye, as occurs when there is a lesion of the optic nerve between the retina and the optic chiasm, or severe retinal disease.

4. Test the **eye movements** (see Fig 8.2).

5. Look also for fatigability of eye muscles by asking the patient to look up at a hatpin or finger for about half a minute. In myasthenia gravis the muscles tire and the eyelids begin to droop.

6. Test **colour vision** if acuity is not poor. You can use Ishihara test plates (where coloured spots form numbers). Red desaturation (impaired ability to see red objects) can occur with optic nerve disease. Red–green colour blindness affects 7% of males (X-linked recessive).

7. Test the **corneal reflex**, if indicated (p. 196).

Consider the possibility that the patient may have a glass eye. This should be suspected if visual acuity is zero in one eye and no pupillary reaction is apparent.[1]

---

1 Attempts to examine and interpret the fundus of a glass eye will amuse the patient but are always unsuccessful.

HORNER'S SYNDROME

Interruption of the sympathetic innervation of the eye at any point results in **Horner's syndrome**. This causes:

- **partial ptosis** (as sympathetic fibres supply the smooth muscle of both eyelids)
- a **constricted pupil** (because of an unbalanced parasympathetic action), which reacts normally to light.

There may be reduced sweating on the forehead on the affected side (anhydrosis). Note that perceptible anisocoria (inequality of the diameters of the pupils) is found in 20% of people. Its presence should not always cause alarm.

T&O'C examination hint box

Elderly people quite often have imperceptible pupillary light reactions.

OPHTHALMOSCOPY

Successful ophthalmoscopy requires considerable practice. It is important that it be performed in a darkened room so that the patient's pupils are at least partly dilated and you are not distracted. It can be easier to perform the examination, especially of the fundi, through the patient's spectacles. Otherwise, the patient's refractive error should be corrected by use of the appropriate ophthalmoscope lens. The patient should be asked to stare at a point on the opposite wall or on the ceiling and to ignore the light of the ophthalmoscope. Patients will often attempt to focus on the ophthalmoscope light and should be asked not to do this initially.

1. Begin by examining the **cornea**. Use your right eye to examine the patient's right eye, and vice versa. Turn the ophthalmoscope lens to +20 and examine the cornea from about 20 cm away from the patient. Look particularly for corneal ulceration. Turn the lens gradually down to 0 while moving closer to the patient. Structures, including the **lens**, **humour** and then the retina at increasing distance into the eye, will swim into focus.

2. Examine the **retina**. Focus on one of the retinal arteries and follow it into the optic disc. The **normal optic disc** is

round and paler than the surrounding retina. The margin of the disc is usually sharply outlined but will appear blurred if there is papilloedema or papillitis, or pale if there is optic atrophy. Inspect the rest of the retina and especially look for the retinal changes of diabetes mellitus or hypertension.

- There are two main types of retinal change in **diabetes mellitus**: non-proliferative and proliferative.
  - Non-proliferative changes include: (1) two types of haemorrhages—**dot haemorrhages**, which occur in the inner retinal layers, and **blot haemorrhages**, which are larger and occur more superficially in the nerve fibre layer; (2) **microaneurysms** (tiny bulges in the vessel wall), which are due to vessel wall damage; and (3) two types of exudates—**hard exudates**, which have straight edges and are due to leakage of protein from damaged arteriolar walls, and **soft exudates** (cottonwool spots), which have a fluffy appearance and are due to microinfarcts (see Fig 8.3).
  - Proliferative changes include new vessel formation, which can lead to retinal detachment or vitreous haemorrhage.

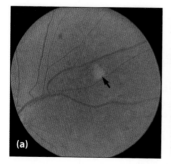 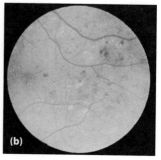

Figure 8.3 Diabetic retinopathy. **(a)** Soft exudate (arrow) and small haemorrhages. **(b)** Microaneurysms (dots), retinal haemorrhages (blots) and hard yellow exudates. (Dr Chris Kennedy and Professor Ian Constable, Lions Eye Institute, Perth.)

- **Hypertensive** changes can be classified from grades 1 to 4:
  - **grade 1**—'silver wiring' of the arteries only (sclerosis of the vessel wall reduces its transparency so that the central light streak becomes broader and shinier)
  - **grade 2**—silver wiring of the arteries plus arteriovenous nipping or nicking (indentation or deflection of the veins where they are crossed by the arteries)
  - **grade 3**—grade 2 plus haemorrhages (flame-shaped) and exudates (soft—cottonwool spots due to ischaemia; or hard—lipid residues from leaking vessels)
  - **grade 4**—grade 3 changes plus papilloedema (see Fig 8.4).

  It is important to describe the changes present rather than just give a grade.
3. Inspect carefully for **central retinal artery occlusion**, where the whole fundus appears milky-white because of retinal oedema and the arteries become greatly reduced in diameter.

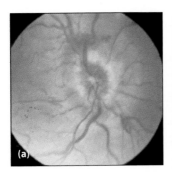 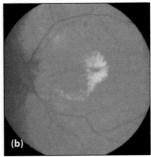

Figure 8.4 Fundoscopy. **(a)** Papilloedema. **(b)** Grade 4 hypertensive retinopathy, with papilloedema, a 'macular star' of hard exudates collecting around the fovea and retinal oedema. (Courtesy of Lions Eye Institute.)

4. **Central retinal vein thrombosis** causes tortuous retinal veins and haemorrhages scattered over the whole retina, particularly occurring alongside the veins.
5. **Retinitis pigmentosa** causes a scattering of black pigment in a criss-cross pattern. This will be missed if the periphery of the retina is not examined.
6. Finally, ask the patient to look directly at the light. This allows you to locate and inspect the **macula** (an oval, yellow spot near the centre of the retina that is important for central vision).

The ears

EXAMINATION ANATOMY

The pinna, external auditory canal and eardrum (see Fig 8.5) are easily assessed with simple equipment. Tests of hearing can also provide information about the severity and anatomical site of hearing loss.

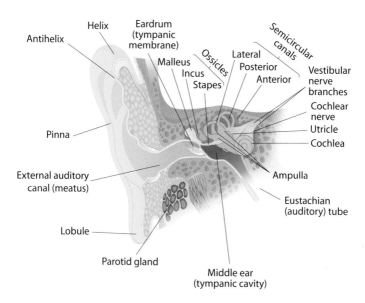

Figure 8.5 Cross-sectional anatomy of the ear showing the pinna, external auditory canal, middle and inner ear.

EXAMINATION METHOD

Ear examination consists of inspection and palpation, auriscopic examination and hearing testing.

1. Inspect the position of the **pinna** and note its size and shape. Note any scars or swelling around the ears. Look for:
   - an obvious accessory auricle (separate piece of cartilage away from the pinna), cauliflower ears (haematomas from recurrent trauma, which fill in the hollows of the ear) and bat ears (protrusion of the ears from the side of the head)
   - signs of **inflammation**, including gouty tophi (nodular, firm, pale and non-tender chalky depositions of urate in the cartilage of the ear, specific but not sensitive for gout)
   - any obvious **ear discharge**—if there is a discharge, note its colour, translucency and consistency.
2. Palpate the pinna for swelling or nodules. Pull down the pinna gently; infection of the external canal often causes tenderness of the pinna.

T&O'C examination hint box

Choose the largest speculum that the auditory meatus will allow. Typically a speculum with a 4-mm tip will suit adults and a 2-mm tip will suit children.

---

3. **Auriscopic examination** of the ears requires use of an earpiece that fits comfortably in the ear canal to allow inspection of the ear canal and tympanic membrane. This examination is essential if there is a history of recent deafness or a painful ear and for the patient who has had a head injury. Always examine both ears!
   - The correct technique is as follows (see Fig 8.6).
     - Ask the patient to turn his or her head slightly to the side.
     - Pull the pinna up, out and back to straighten the ear canal and provide optimal vision.
     - Stretch out the fingers of your hand holding the auriscope to touch the patient's cheek, to steady the

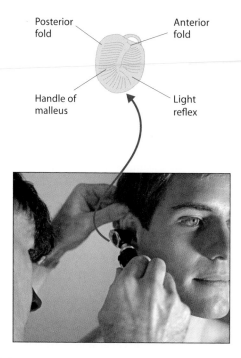

Figure 8.6 Use of the auriscope.

instrument and prevent sudden movements of the patient's head.

– When examining the patient's right ear, hold the auriscope preferably in a downward position with your right hand, while using your left hand to pull the pinna. An alternative position involves holding the auriscope upwards, but there is a risk that if the patient moves suddenly injury is more likely to occur.

• Look at the **external canal** for:

– any evidence of inflammation (e.g. redness or swelling) or discharge; there should be no tenderness unless there is inflammation

- ear **wax** (cerumen), which is white or yellowish, and translucent and shiny; it may obscure the view of the tympanic membrane
- blood or cerebrospinal fluid (watery, clear fluid), which may be seen in the canal if there is a fracture at the base of the skull
- vesicles (fluid-filled blisters) on the posterior wall around the external auditory meatus in patients with herpes zoster.

- Inspect the **tympanic membrane** (eardrum) by introducing the speculum further into the canal in a forward but downward direction. The normal tympanic membrane is greyish and reflects light from the centre at approximately 5 or 7 o'clock. Note:
  - colour
  - transparency
  - any evidence of dilated blood vessels
  - bulging or retraction (bulging can suggest underlying fluid or pus in the middle ear)
  - any perforation of the tympanic membrane.

- If a middle ear infection is suspected, **pneumatic auriscopy** can be useful. Use a speculum large enough to occlude the external canal snugly. Attach a rubber squeeze bulb to the auriscope. When the bulb is squeezed gently, air pressure in the canal is increased and the tympanic membrane should move promptly inwards. Absence of, or a decrease in, movement is a sign of fluid in the middle ear.

4. To **test hearing**, whisper numbers 60 cm away from one of the patient's ears while distracting the other ear by movement of your finger in the auditory canal. Then repeat the process with the other ear. With practice the normal range of hearing will be appreciated. Then perform Rinné's and Weber's tests:

- **Rinné's test:** place the base of a vibrating 256-Hz tuning fork on the mastoid process. When the sound is no longer heard, move the tines of the fork close to the auditory meatus where, if air conduction is (as is normal) better than bone conduction, it will again be audible.

- **Weber's test:** place a vibrating 256-Hz fork base at the centre of the patient's forehead. Nerve deafness causes the sound to be heard better in the normal ear, but with conduction deafness the sound is better heard in the 'abnormal' ear.

The nose

EXAMINATION METHOD

Nose examination consists of inspection, palpation and testing sense of smell.

1. Inspect the skin. Note any **nasal deviation** (best seen from behind the patient looking down). Note any periorbital swelling (e.g. from sinusitis). Inspect the nares by pressing the tip of the nose upwards with your thumb.
2. Palpate the nasal bones, then feel for facial swelling or signs of inflammation. Block each nostril to assess any obstruction by asking the patient to inhale.
3. Tilt the patient's head back and look into the nose with a torch. A speculum can be used to open the nares. Look at the mucosa for discolouration and for discharge and deviation of the nasal septum (see Fig 8.7).
4. If there is a history of **anosmia** (loss of smell), test smell (cranial nerve I; p. 188).

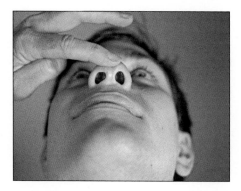

Figure 8.7   Examining the nasal mucosa and septum.

The mouth and throat

EXAMINATION ANATOMY

See Figure 8.8.

EXAMINATION METHOD

Throat examination consists of inspection and palpation.

1. Look in turn at the lips, buccal mucosa, gums, palate and teeth.
   - Note any signs of **inflammation** (e.g. redness, swelling).
   - Inspect the **tongue** first in the mouth, then ask the patient to poke it out, and then ask the patient to touch it to the roof of the mouth (to look at the floor of the mouth).
   - Ask the patient to say 'Aaah' and inspect the **oropharynx** and **uvula** (you often need to press a tongue depressor on the posterior tongue to see properly).

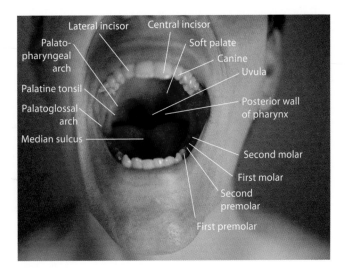

Figure 8.8 The mouth and throat.

- Inspect the **tonsils** (note the size, shape, colour, discharge or membrane—they involute in adults and may not be seen).
2. Palpate the tongue for **lumps** (wear gloves). Palpate the **salivary glands** (p. 145). Finally, examine the **cervical lymph nodes** (p. 175).

T&O'C examination essentials

The mouth and throat are the gate and entry to the gut and the lungs. Look (and smell) for:
- peridental inflammation
- gingivitis
- poor dentition
- leucoplakia
- tongue fissures
- oral cancers
- fasciculations
- fetor hepaticus.

The eyes, ears, nose and throat OSCE: hints panel

1. Examine this patient's sclerae and conjunctivae. (Wash your hands)
   (a) Stand back to look. This is probably a spot diagnosis.
   (b) Look for scleral icterus. Proceed accordingly if present to examine for signs of chronic liver disease.
   (c) Note the distribution of any redness (e.g. single red eye in iritis). Decide whether conjunctival redness (injection) is central (iritis) or spares the central region (conjunctivitis).
   (d) If there is conjunctival injection, ask for gloves before pulling the lower lid down. Note any ocular discharge (conjunctivitis).
   (e) If there is pallor, pull down the lower lid and compare the pearly white posterior part of the conjunctiva with the red anterior part.
   (f) If there is chemosis, look for proptosis and other signs of thyrotoxicosis.
   (g) Look at the iris (haziness indicates oedema or inflammation).
   (h) Look at and test the pupils (e.g. small irregular pupil in iritis; dilated, oval, poorly reactive pupil in acute glaucoma).
   (i) Assess eye movement (painful in scleritis).
   (j) Perform fundoscopy.
   (k) Look for systemic evidence of vasculitis (e.g. urinalysis).
   (l) Synthesise and present your findings.

2. Look in this patient's fundi.
   (Wash your hands)
   (a) The pupils will probably have been dilated.
   (b) Use the ophthalmoscope in the approved manner.
   (c) Look particularly for changes of hypertension or diabetes.
   (d) Synthesise and present your findings.
3. This woman has experienced sudden loss of vision in one eye.
   Please examine her.
   (Wash your hands)
   (a) Test *each* eye for visual acuity and fully assess the visual
       fields.
   (b) Assess each pupil's reaction to light and accommodation,
       and for an afferent pupillary defect (optic nerve damage).
   (c) Test eye movement and ask about any pain on movement
       (optic neuritis).
   (d) Examine the fundi. Note whether the disc is swollen and is
       abnormally pink or white (ischaemic optic neuropathy). Note
       any retinal fundal pallor (arterial occlusion), haemorrhages
       (venous occlusion) or an obvious embolus (at an arterial
       bifurcation).
   (e) Test colour vision if red–green test plates are available (for
       optic nerve damage).
   (f) Auscultate for a carotid bruit (stenosis).
   (g) Take her pulse (atrial fibrillation) and blood pressure
       (hypertension).
   (h) Ask whether you may test the patient's urine for blood or
       protein (vasculitis).
   (i) Synthesise and present your findings.
4. This man complains of a sore ear. Examine his auditory canal
   and ear drum.
   (Wash your hands)
   (a) Note whether he looks unwell or feverish.
   (b) Look at the pinna and external auditory meatus for gouty
       tophi, dermatitis, cellulitis, signs of trauma (e.g. haematoma),
       scars (e.g. surgery) and discharge. Look at *both* ears.
   (c) Ask the patient whether the ear is painful before using the
       auriscope to examine the canal and drum.
   (d) Look for erythema or blisters in the canal, and for wax, pus
       or discharge from the drum.
   (e) Inspect the tympanic membrane (ear drum) for perforation,
       grommets (tympanostomy tubes) or loss of the normal shiny
       appearance.
   (f) Test hearing and perform Rinné's and Weber's tests.
   (g) Palpate the temporomandibular joint for tenderness and
       crepitus (referred pain).
   (h) Examine the throat for inflammation (referred pain).
   (i) Synthesise and present your findings.

5. This patient complains of recurrent sore throat. Please examine her.

   (Wash your hands and don gloves)

   (a) Remove dentures if the patient wears them.[2] Note any drooling or flushing, and whether she appears ill.

   (b) Take a torch and ask the patient to open wide.

   (c) Inspect her mouth and pharynx using a tongue depressor. Note tonsillar enlargement and any erythema or other signs of inflammation.

   (d) Note whether the patient cannot open her mouth fully (trismus)—lockjaw is reduced jaw opening that can occur in tetanus.

   (e) Feel the oral cavity and tongue gently with a gloved finger.

   (f) Palpate the cervical nodes carefully.

   (g) Take her temperature (fever).

   (h) Synthesise and present your findings.

T&O'C examination essentials

The eyes, ears, nose and throat

1. Important local and systemic disease can be missed unless the eyes are examined as part of a general medical examination.

2. Accurate fundoscopy with the ophthalmoscope requires practice. Dilating the patient's pupils may be necessary to obtain an adequate view.

3. Subtle eye signs, such as Horner's syndrome, will be missed unless time is taken to stand back and compare the two sides.

4. Complete examination of the mouth and throat includes palpating the draining lymph nodes (cervical nodes).

---

2 Remember where you put them down; do not lose them.

The thyroid and endocrine system

Remember, however, that every patient upon whom you wait will examine you critically and form an estimate of you by the way in which you conduct yourself at the bedside. Skill and nicety in manipulation, whether in the simple act of feeling the pulse or in the performance of any minor operation will do more towards establishing confidence in you, than a string of diplomas, or the reputation of extensive hospital experience.

Sir William Osler (1849–1919)

The thyroid

PRESENTING SYMPTOMS

The thyroid is a small gland that is usually unobtrusive but exerts a powerful influence on all parts of the body. Under- or over-activity produces characteristic symptoms and signs:

- **Thyrotoxicosis** (excess thyroid hormone production) can cause a preference for cooler weather, weight loss, increased appetite (polyphagia), palpitations (sinus tachycardia or atrial fibrillation), increased sweating, nervousness, irritability, diarrhoea, amenorrhoea, muscle weakness and exertional dyspnoea.

- **Hypothyroidism** (myxoedema—decreased thyroid hormone production) can result in a preference for warmer weather, weight gain, lethargy, swelling of the eyelids (oedema), hoarse voice, constipation and coarse dry skin.

THE HISTORY

Find out about previous surgery (e.g. thyroidectomy) and about other treatments for thyroid disease, such as radioiodine, anti-thyroid drugs, thyroid replacement treatment (thyroxine) or use of the drug amiodarone (this antiarrhythmic drug contains iodine and can cause hyper- or hypothyroidism). Many endocrine conditions are chronic and their effect on a patient's ability to work and look after him- or herself must be assessed. There may be a history in the family of thyroid conditions. Find out where the patient grew up (there are areas of endemic goitre caused by iodine deficiency).

EXAMINATION ANATOMY

The word thyroid comes from the Greek *thyreoeides*, meaning shield-shaped. It sits like a shield in the front of the neck (see Fig 9.1). Its two lobes are connected by an isthmus, which lies just below the larynx. It may be palpable in thin people.

THYROTOXICOSIS

Examine a suspected case of thyrotoxicosis as follows.

1. Look for signs of weight loss, anxiety and the frightened facies of the thyrotoxic (see Fig 9.2).
2. Ask the patient to put out his or her arms and look for a **fine tremor**.
3. Look at the patient's nails for **onycholysis** (Plummer's nails—separation of the distal nail from the nail bed) and for thyroid acropachy (clubbing).
4. Inspect for **palmar erythema** (a red appearance of the outer parts of the palms) and feel the palms for warmth and sweatiness (from sympathetic over-activity).
5. Take the patient's **pulse**. Note the presence of sinus tachycardia or atrial fibrillation. The pulse may also have a collapsing character due to a high cardiac output.

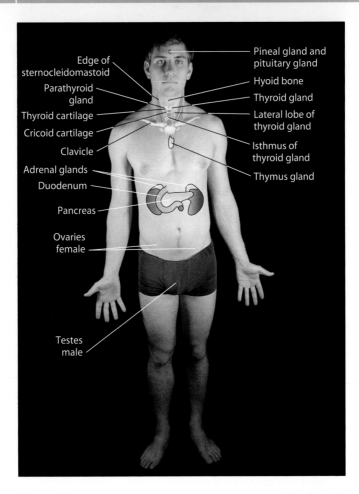

Figure 9.1   Surface anatomy of the neck and thyroid and the sites of the endocrine glands.

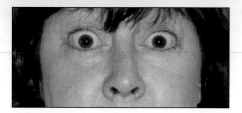

Figure 9.2 Thyrotoxicosis: thyroid stare and exophthalmos.
(Kryger, MH. *Atlas of Clinical Sleep Medicine* 2014; 25(11), Figure 15.1.1b.)

6. Test for **proximal myopathy** (weakness of the muscles at the shoulders and hips) and tap the arm reflexes for abnormal briskness, especially in the relaxation phase.
7. Examine the **eyes**.
    - Look for **exophthalmos** (protrusion of the eyeball out of the orbit).
    - Then examine for **lid retraction**, which is suggested by a widened palpebral fissure.
    - Test for **lid lag** by watching for lagging of the descent of the upper lid as the patient follows your finger while you move it at moderate speed from the upper to the lower part of the visual field.
    - Then stand behind the patient and look over the forehead to assess for the degree of **proptosis**, which is actual protrusion of the globes from the orbits.
    - Next look for the complications of proptosis:
        - chemosis (oedema of the conjunctivae)
        - conjunctivitis (inflammation of the conjunctivae)
        - corneal ulceration (it may be necessary to stain the cornea with fluorescein)
        - optic atrophy (rare—pallor of the optic disc when examined with the ophthalmoscope, and due to ischaemia of the retina from stretching in exophthalmos)
        - ophthalmoplegia (upward gaze tends to be lost first, and later convergence is weakened).
8. Examine for thyroid enlargement (see p. 248). A thrill may be present over the gland on palpation. Listen over the gland for a bruit.

9. Examine the **heart** for systolic flow murmurs and for signs of cardiac failure (see Ch 4).

10. Look for **pretibial myxoedema** (bilateral firm and elevated nodules and plaques on the shins, which may be pink or brown).

11. Test for **hyper-reflexia** in the legs.

HYPOTHYROIDISM

Examine the patient with suspected hypothyroidism as follows.

1. A variable number of the following signs may be present. Look for signs of obvious mental and physical **sluggishness**. Note peripheral cyanosis, a cool and dry skin and the yellow skin discolouration of hypercarotenaemia (a result of reduced metabolism of carotene).

2. Take the patient's **pulse**, which may be of small volume and slow.

3. Test for **median nerve entrapment** (carpal tunnel syndrome). *Phalen's sign* (tingling in the median nerve distribution during prolonged extension of the wrist) and *Tinel's sign* (tapping over the flexor retinaculum causing paraesthesia in the tendon sheath when the test is positive) have limited diagnostic value.

4. Look at the patient's **face**. The skin, but not the sclera, may appear yellow due to hypercarotenaemia. The skin may be generally thickened, and **alopecia** (loss of hair) may be present, as may **vitiligo** (an associated autoimmune disease).

5. Inspect the **eyes** for periorbital oedema and xanthelasma and note loss or thinning of the outer third of the eyebrows.

6. Ask the patient to speak, and listen for **coarse, croaking, slow speech**.

7. Test for a **'hung up' ankle reflex** with the patient kneeling on a chair (the foot plantarflexes normally when the Achilles tendon is tapped, but then dorsiflexes much more slowly; see Fig 9.3).

EXAMINATION OF THE THYROID

The thyroid should be examined by inspection, palpation, percussion and auscultation.

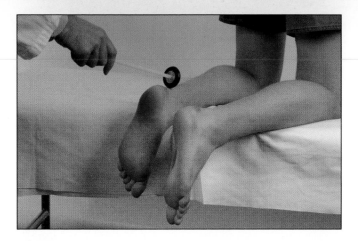

Figure 9.3 Testing ankle jerks. This method best demonstrates the 'hung up' reflexes of hypothyroidism. Look for rapid dorsiflexion followed by slow plantar flexion after the tendon is tapped. (Courtesy of Glenn McCulloch.)

Inspection

Sometimes the isthmus of the normal thyroid is visible as a diffuse central swelling in the neck. Enlargement of the gland, called a **goitre**, should be apparent on inspection.

1. Look at the front and sides of the neck and decide whether there is localised or general swelling of the gland.
2. Then ask the patient to **swallow a sip of water** while you watch the swelling. Only a goitre or a **thyroglossal cyst** will rise during swallowing, because of their attachment to the larynx.
3. Ask the patient to **stick out his or her tongue**: a thyroglossal cyst will move up, but a goitre will not.
4. Inspect the skin of the neck for scars and look for prominent veins (suggesting thoracic inlet obstruction caused by a retrosternal thyroid mass).

Palpation

1. Systematically feel both lobes of the gland and its isthmus from behind the patient using the tips of your fingers (see Fig 9.4). Note the size, shape, consistency, symmetry,

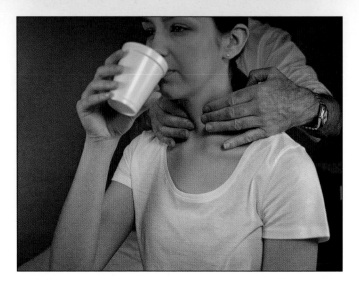

Figure 9.4 Examination of the thyroid.

tenderness and mobility of the gland and the presence of a thrill. Decide whether the lower limit of the gland is palpable.

2. Ask the patient to swallow and feel for the swelling to rise.
3. Feel next for the cervical lymph nodes (p. 145).

Percussion

1. Percuss over the upper sternum. Dullness may indicate a retrosternal goitre.
2. Test for **Pemberton's sign**. Ask the patient to lift up both arms as high as possible. In thoracic inlet obstruction (e.g. by a retrosternal goitre), the patient's face will turn red, cyanosis will occur, the neck veins will swell and stridor (harsh inspiration caused by a partly occluded upper airway) may occur.

Auscultation

1. Auscultate over the gland. A soft bruit may be audible when an overactive gland is very vascular.
2. Listen to the patient's breathing for stridor.

3. If there is a goitre, apply mild compression to the lateral lobes and listen again for stridor.

DIABETES MELLITUS

In patients with diabetes mellitus, you need to assess carefully for complications that are often multi-system. One approach is as follows:

1. **General inspection.**
   - Look for signs of dehydration.
   - Weigh the patient (obesity).
   - Note the patient's mental state (coma can occur).
   - There may be signs of Cushing's syndrome or acromegaly (secondary causes of diabetes mellitus).
2. **Lower limbs.**
   - Look at the skin on the patient's legs for leg ulcers, skin infections (e.g. boils) or pigmented scars. **Necrobiosis lipoidica diabeticorum** is a rare scarred lesion with a red margin and yellow centre that is usually found on the shins.
   - Note any insulin injection site changes (causing fat atrophy or hypertrophy).
   - Note any oedema.
   - Examine for **neurological disease in the legs** (e.g. peripheral neuropathy, loss of proximal muscle power).
   - Examine for loss of the peripheral pulses.
   - Feel the temperature of the feet (**peripheral vascular disease**).
3. **The face.**
   - Examine the patient's eyes. The fundi in particular need careful assessment for diabetic retinopathy (p. 233).
   - Other signs can include a diabetic third cranial nerve palsy (typically with pupil sparing).
4. **The ears, nose and throat.**
   - Look for any evidence of infection (e.g. fungal).
   - Examine for a carotid bruit (carotid stenosis).
5. **The chest and abdomen.**
   - Look for signs of infection.
   - Palpate for hepatomegaly (fatty liver).

6. **Urinalysis.** Test for glucose and protein.
7. **Blood pressure.** Measure for postural hypotension (autonomic neuropathy).

The endocrine system: a systematic approach

Endocrine diseases can affect multiple organ systems. Some of the signs linked to the more important endocrine diseases are summarised here.

1. Pick up the patient's hands. Look at their overall size (increased in acromegaly—excess growth hormone) and for abnormalities of the nails (hyperthyroidism and hypothyroidism).
2. Take the patient's pulse (thyroid disease) and blood pressure (hypertension in Cushing's syndrome (glucocorticoid excess) or postural hypotension in Addison's disease (adrenocortical hypofunction).
3. Look for Trousseau's sign (tetany from hypocalcaemia in hypoparathyroidism). Inflate the blood pressure cuff above systolic and wait 2 minutes: if positive, the thumb becomes adducted and the fingers extended.
4. Go to the axillae. Look for loss of axillary hair (pituitary failure: pan-hypopituitarism) or acanthosis nigricans and skin tags (acromegaly).
5. Examine the patient's eyes (hyperthyroidism) and the fundi (diabetes mellitus). Look at the face for hirsutism or fine-wrinkled hairless skin (pan-hypopituitarism). Note any skin greasiness, acne or plethora (Cushing's syndrome; see Table 3.1).
6. Look at the mouth for protrusion of the chin and enlargement of the tongue (acromegaly; see Table 3.1) or buccal pigmentation (Addison's disease).
7. Examine the neck for thyroid enlargement. Palpate for supraclavicular fat pads (Cushing's syndrome).
8. Inspect the chest wall for hirsutism or loss of body hair, reduction in breast size in women (pan-hypopituitarism). Look for gynaecomastia in men (e.g. testicular failure, thyrotoxicosis). Look for nipple pigmentation (Addison's disease).

9. Examine the abdomen for hirsutism, central fat deposition and purple striae (Cushing's syndrome).
10. Look at the legs for diabetic changes, including:
    - loss of peripheral pulses
    - signs of limb ischaemia
    - peripheral neuropathy
    - Charcot's joints
    - arterial ulcers
    - necrobiosis lipoidica diabeticorum
    - insulin injection sites
    - fat atrophy.
11. Test the urine (diabetes mellitus).

The endocrine OSCE: hints panel

1. This woman has had thyrotoxicosis. Take a history from her.
   (a) Ask her the following:
       (i) How long is it since you became unwell?
       (ii) Do you feel back to normal now? How has the illness affected your life and work?
       (iii) Have you lost weight during this illness? If so, how much?
       (iv) Have you found hot weather more uncomfortable than usual? Have you felt more anxious than before?
       (v) Have you had problems with diarrhoea?
       (vi) Have you had heart palpitations? How often? Were they regular or irregular?
       (vii) Have you had a goitre?
       (viii) Have you had problems with your eyes? What has happened to them? Has this improved?
       (ix) Is there thyroid trouble in your family?
       (x) What treatments have you had? Have you had to stop any medications because of problems?
   (b) Synthesise and present your findings.
2. This man has been diagnosed with hypothyroidism. Take a history from him.
   (a) Ask him the following:
       (i) How long have you been unwell?
       (ii) Do you feel back to normal now? How has the illness affected your life and work?
       (iii) Have you put on weight? If so, how much?
       (iv) Have you found cold weather more intolerable than usual?
       (v) Have you had problems with constipation?
       (vi) Have you had a goitre?

       (vii) Is there thyroid trouble in your family?

      (viii) What treatments have you had? Did you have to stop any of your previous medications because of problems?

  (b) Synthesise and present your findings.

3. Please examine the eyes of this woman with thyrotoxicosis. (Wash your hands)

  (a) Stand back to look for general abnormalities (tremor, apparent loss of weight, thyroid stare and the presence of a goitre).

  (b) Look at the patient's eyes from in front and from above (looking over the forehead) for proptosis.

  (c) Look at the conjunctivae for chemosis.

  (d) Test for lid lag.

  (e) Look for chemosis, conjunctivitis and corneal ulceration.

  (f) Examine the fundi for optic atrophy if exophthalmos is present.

  (g) Examine her eye movements in full.

  (h) Synthesise and present your findings.

4. Please take an appropriate history from this man who has had type 2 diabetes mellitus for 20 years.

  (a) Ask him the following:

      (i) How was your diabetes first diagnosed?

      (ii) What has happened to your weight since then?

     (iii) What type of diet are you on? Do you understand the reason for this type of diet?

     (iv) What medicines do you take for diabetes?

      (v) Are you using insulin? Tell me about your usual regimen and how you make adjustments to your dose.

     (vi) Have you had hypoglycaemic episodes?

    (vii) How often do you test your blood sugar? Do you keep a record of your results? Has your sugar control been good?

    (viii) Have you had any problems with your vision? Do you have your eyes checked regularly? What have you been told about any complications involving your eyes?

     (ix) Have you had any kidney problems?

     (x) Have you been told that you might have vascular problems involving the heart or be at risk of stroke?

     (xi) Do you smoke? Do you know what your cholesterol level is?

    (xii) Have you had any problems with dizziness on standing?

    (xiii) Have you had any problems with your digestion?

    (xiv) Have you had numbness in your fingers or toes?

    (xv) Have you had problems with ulcers on your legs that are slow to heal?

    (xvi) Have you had problems with skin or urinary infections?

  (b) Synthesise and present your findings.

T&O'C examination essentials

The endocrine system

1. Not all patients with thyroid disease will have a goitre but careful examination of the neck for the presence of a goitre is part of the routine physical examination.

2. A thyroid that lies higher in the neck than average may appear enlarged but when it is not prominent enough to be palpable there is unlikely to be a goitre.

3. Thyroid disease causes systemic symptoms and signs that are often of an insidious onset and may not be noticed by the patient or the patient's relatives.

4. Diabetics should be well informed about the complications of their disease. Every opportunity should be taken to remind them of the importance of careful blood sugar control and cardiovascular risk factor control.

5. Develop your own system for the complete examination of the diabetic patient.

6. Skin hyperpigmentation (e.g. in the palmar creases) is a sign of Addison's disease (adrenocortical failure). Check these patients for orthostatic hypotension.

The breasts

Variability is the law of life, and as no two faces are the same, so no two bodies are alike, and no two individuals react alike and behave alike under the abnormal conditions which we know as disease.

Sir William Osler (1849–1919)

Breast examination is a routine part of the general physical examination in women.

The history

Ask about the reason for presentation—for example, a routine breast examination, an abnormality that has been noticed (many women regularly examine their breasts for lumps), nipple discharge, breast pain or a request for assessment because of a family history of carcinoma of the breast in first- or second-degree relatives (see Questions box 10.1). Also consider asking about symptoms that may indicate metastatic spread of breast cancer, such as:

- increasing dyspnoea
- bone pain or symptoms of hypercalcaemia (nausea, anorexia, constipation, confusion)
- abdominal pain or swelling, or jaundice
- headache, confusion or weakness.

Questions box 10.1   Questions to ask the woman who presents for a breast examination

! denotes an urgent problem or a high risk

1. Have you noticed a lump?
2. If so, is it painful? (Rarely are malignant lumps painful, except for the rare inflammatory carcinoma)
3. Has it appeared just before menstruation? (These are often hormonal and benign, but must be examined)
! 4. Have you had breast cancer before? (A strong risk factor)
5. Is there a history of breast cancer in your family? (Breast carcinoma in two first-degree female relatives or one first-degree male relative, or bilateral breast cancer in one first-degree relative, is an important risk factor for breast cancer)
! 6. Have you been tested for the breast cancer gene? (Women who are BRCA1 or BRCA2 positive have a 70% chance of developing breast cancer and a 50% chance of developing ovarian cancer)
7. Have you had a previous breast biopsy? (The biopsied area may feel firm or lumpy; a previous biopsy may have shown atypical ductal hyperplasia, which is considered a premalignant condition)
8. Also ask about other factors that can influence risk:
   - At what age did you begin to have periods? (Menarche)
   - Have you stopped having periods?
   - How old were you when you had your first full-term pregnancy?
   - Did you breastfeed your child(ren)?
   - Have you used the contraceptive pill?

Examination of the breasts

Male doctors (and students) should have a chaperone.

INSPECTION

1. Ask the patient to sit up with her chest fully exposed.
2. Look at the nipples for retraction (due to **cancer** or fibrosis; note in some patients retraction may be normal) and **Paget's disease** of the nipple (where underlying breast cancer causes a unilateral red, scaling or bleeding area).
3. Inspect the rest of the skin. Look for **visible veins** (which, if unilateral, suggest a cancer), skin **dimpling** and peau d'orange skin (where advanced breast cancer causes oedematous skin pitted by the sweat glands).

4. Ask the patient to **raise her arms above her head**. Look for tethering of the nipples or skin, a shift in the relative position of the nipples or a fixed mass distorting the breast. Look for axillary lumps.

5. Ask the patient to rest her hands on her hips and then press her hands against her hips (the **pectoral contraction manoeuvre**). This accentuates areas of dimpling or fixation.

PALPATION

1. Make sure your hands are clean and warm.

2. Ask the patient to lie down. It can be helpful to have her place her hand, for the same side (ipsilateral), behind her head. The presence of breast implants makes the examination much more difficult: in this case, the patient's ipsilateral arm should be kept down at her side and the breast examined while she lies supine.

3. Feel each breast systematically (see Figs 10.1 and 10.2).

4. Next, feel **behind the nipple** for lumps and note whether any **fluid** can be expressed: bright blood (e.g. from a duct papilloma or, more rarely, a carcinoma), yellow serous fluid (e.g. fibroadenosis), serous fluid (e.g. early pregnancy), milky fluid (e.g. lactation) or green fluid (e.g. mammary duct ectasia).

5. Examine both the **supraclavicular** and **axillary** regions for lymphadenopathy (p. 175).

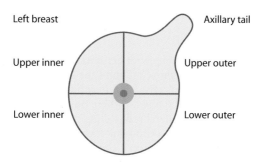

Figure 10.1 Quadrants of the breast.

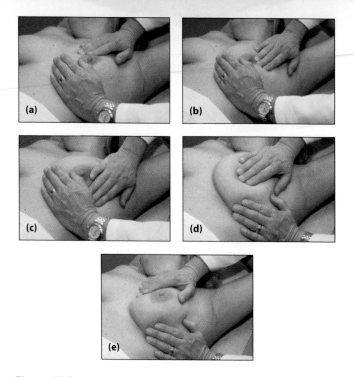

Figure 10.2   Palpating the breasts. **(a)–(e)** The patient is placed in the supine position, and the ipsilateral arm is extended above her head. The examiner palpates the breast with his or her flattened fingers against the chest wall. Palpation begins at the sternum and continues in a lateral direction until the mid-axillary line is passed. Use the pulps of your three middle fingers. Think of the breast like a clock face and palpate each 'hour' of the clock, covering all of the breast in turn from the clavicle above to the lower rib cage below. The nipples and areolar areas are separately compressed. (Baggish MS, Karram MM. *Atlas of Pelvic Anatomy and Gynecologic Surgery 3e*. Elsevier; 2011 Figure 105.13).

EVALUATION OF A BREAST LUMP

1. The following points need to be carefully elucidated if a lump is detected.
   - *Position:* the breast quadrant involved and proximity to the nipple.

- *Size, shape and consistency:* a hard, irregular nodule is characteristic of carcinoma. A firm, round mobile lump suggests a fibroadenoma.
- *Tenderness:* suggests an inflammatory or cystic lesion; breast cancer is usually not tender.
- *Fixation:* mobility is determined by taking the breast between the hands and moving it over the chest wall with the arm relaxed and then with the hand pressing on the hip (to tense the pectoralis major). For lower outer quadrant lesions, the arm should push against a wall in front of the patient (to tense the serratus anterior muscle). In advanced carcinoma the lump may be fixed to the chest wall.
- *Single or multiple lesions:* multiple nodules suggest benign cystic disease or fibroadenosis.
- *Lymph node enlargement:* examine the **draining** axillary and supraclavicular lymph nodes—the presence of nodes suggests metastatic disease.

2. If carcinoma is suspected, examine for metastatic disease. Examine for a pleural effusion. Check for vertebral or other bony tenderness. Palpate for a hard, irregular liver (malignant hepatomegaly).

THE MALE BREASTS

In men with true gynaecomastia (breast tissue enlargement), a disc of breast tissue can be palpated under the areola. This is not present in men who are merely obese.

T&O'C examination essentials

Breast examination
1. A careful history can give important information about risk. This is a common OSCE topic.
2. Examination of the female breasts is a routine aspect of physical examination of a woman.
3. The examination is not complete unless the draining lymph nodes are also examined.
4. Examine for evidence of distant metastases if carcinoma is suspected.
5. The most common cause of true male breast enlargement (and tenderness) is use of the drug spironolactone—usually for the treatment of heart failure.

The joints

*The greater the ignorance the greater the
dogmatism.*

Sir William Osler (1849–1919)

Joint abnormalities are commonly due to injury, inflammation
or degeneration (wear and tear). Inflammatory joint conditions
are often associated with abnormalities of the skin and connective tissues.

The rheumatological history

PRESENTING SYMPTOMS (see Box 11.1)

Joint pain and swelling

1. Ask the patient what joint problems have occurred.
   Arthralgia refers to joint pain without swelling, whereas
   arthritis means both pain and swelling.
2. Determine whether:
   - one or many joints are involved
   - the changes are symmetrical
   - symptoms are of an acute or a chronic nature
   - the symptoms are getting better or worse.

Patients with rheumatoid arthritis have **joint symptoms
that are worse after rest**, whereas those with osteoarthritis
have **pain that is worse after exercise**.

Box 11.1
Rheumatological history: presenting symptoms

Major symptoms
Joints
Pain
Swelling
Morning stiffness
Loss of function

Back pain
Limb pain

Eyes
Dry eyes and mouth
Red eyes

Raynaud's phenomenon

Systemic and other symptoms
Rash, fever, fatigue, weight loss, diarrhoea, mucosal ulcers

3. Ask about **early morning stiffness**, which is a symptom of active synovitis (inflammation of the synovium).
4. Ask detailed questions about the ability of the patient with arthritis to perform usual activities at home and at work.

Back pain

Back pain is a very common problem. Ask about localisation, whether it is intermittent or progressive, and the relationship to exercise.

- Musculoskeletal pain is characteristically well localised and is aggravated by movement.
- Spinal cord lesions may cause pain that occurs in a dermatomal distribution (see Fig 7.13).
- Osteoporosis (with crush fractures), osteomalacia or infiltration of carcinoma, leukaemia or myeloma may cause progressive and unremitting back pain.
- The pain may be of sudden onset if it results from the crush fracture of a vertebral body.
- **Ankylosing spondylitis** (an inflammatory arthritis of the axial skeleton) causes pain that is usually situated over the sacroiliac joints and lumbar spine and that is improved by exercise; early morning stiffness accompanies the pain.

Limb pain

Ask about past trauma, the distribution of pain and aggravating and relieving factors. Causes of limb pain include:

- musculoskeletal problems (including trauma)
- **polymyalgia rheumatica** (pain and stiffness in the shoulders and hips in patients over the age of 50 years)
- bone disease, such as osteomyelitis, osteomalacia, osteoporosis or tumours
- inflammation of tendons (tenosynovitis), which can produce local pain over the affected area
- vascular disease: consider arterial occlusion if there has been severe pain of sudden onset. Chronic peripheral vascular disease can result in calf pain on exercise that is relieved by rest. This is called *intermittent claudication*. Venous thrombosis can also cause diffuse aching pain in the legs, associated with swelling.

Associated symptoms

- **Dry eyes and mouth.** These are characteristic of Sjögren's syndrome, which is an autoimmune disease. The dry eyes can result in conjunctivitis, keratitis and corneal ulcers.
- **Red eyes.** The seronegative (rheumatoid factor is not present in the blood) spondyloarthropathies and Behçet's syndrome, but not rheumatoid arthritis, may be complicated by iritis (as described on p. 230).
- **Raynaud's phenomenon.** Raynaud's phenomenon is an abnormal vascular response of the exposed fingers (and toes) to cold; the fingers first turn white, then blue and finally become red and painful.
- **Systemic and other symptoms.** Ask about rashes and mucosal ulcers. In patients with back pain, serious spinal pathology should be suspected if there are 'red flag' features (e.g. fever, neurological symptoms or faecal incontinence, weight loss).

PAST HISTORY

Ask about:

- any history of trauma or surgery
- a history of recent infection, including hepatitis, streptococcal pharyngitis, rubella, dysentery (these can be associated with reactive arthritis)

- gonorrhoea or tuberculosis (can cause infective arthritis)
- inflammatory bowel disease causing bloody diarrhoea, which can also result in arthritis
- gout and pseudogout.

SOCIAL HISTORY

Determine the patient's domestic set-up and occupation. This is particularly relevant if a chronic, disabling arthritis has developed.

TREATMENT HISTORY

1. Document current and previous anti-arthritic medications—for example, aspirin, other anti-inflammatory agents (COX-2 selective inhibitors or other NSAIDs), methotrexate, salazopyrin, chloroquine, steroids, anti-tumour necrosis factor (TNF) drugs, glucosamine or other over-the-counter drugs.
2. Ascertain any side effects of these drugs.
3. Enquire about physiotherapy and joint surgery in the past.

FAMILY HISTORY

Some diseases associated with chronic arthritis run in families. For example, rheumatoid arthritis is four times more common in people who have an affected first-degree relative.

Examination anatomy

THE HANDS AND WRISTS

The complex functions of the hand are reflected in the complexity of the wrist and hand joints (see Fig 11.1). The wrist comprises two synovial joints:

- the radiocarpal joint (between the radial head and the proximal carpal bones)
- the midcarpal joint (between the two rows of carpal bones).

Lateral and medial collateral ligaments and anterior and posterior ligaments stabilise the joint surfaces during different movements. Wrist movements include ulnar and lateral deviation, and flexion and extension. A combination of these movements results in circumduction of the hand.

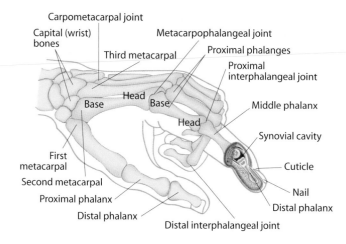

Figure 11.1   Anatomy of the hand and wrist.

The carpometacarpal joints connect the wrist and the hand. These are condyloid synovial joints. Movement can occur around two axes at right angles to each other: flexion and extension, and adduction and abduction. The carpometacarpal joint of the thumb (between the first metacarpal bone and the trapezium) has more complicated articular surfaces. These allow a greater range of movements: flexion, extension, adduction, abduction, rotation and circumduction.

The metacarpophalangeal joints are synovial joints. Possible active movements include flexion, extension, abduction, adduction and some rotation. Extension is much more limited than flexion. The movement of the metacarpophalangeal joint of the thumb is again different. This joint is mostly limited to flexion and extension.

THE KNEES

The knee is the largest hinge joint in the body (see Fig 11.2). It has a large synovium and collateral ligaments to provide lateral stability and cruciate ligaments to limit movement in the antero-posterior direction. Examination of the knee must assess these complicated structures.

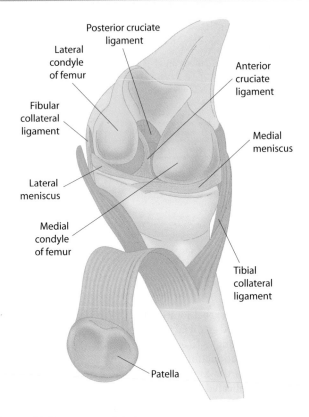

Figure 11.2 Anatomy of the knee.

The rheumatological examination (see

Box 11.2)

GENERAL INSPECTION

A general inspection gives an indication of the patient's functional disability and allows the 'spot diagnosis' of certain conditions.

1. Look at the patient walking into the room and note any apparent pain and difficulty, the posture and whether there is the need for mechanical assistance (walking stick, frame, foot brace etc).

> **Box 11.2**
> **The rheumatological examination sequence**
> 1. General inspection
> 2. Look at all the joints, especially those the history suggests are likely to be abnormal; compare left and right
> 3. Feel the joints and surrounding skin and structures
> 4. Test passive movement, active movement, function and stability
> 5. Measure for fixed deformity

2. Observe the pattern of joint involvement (which joints, and whether symmetrical or not).
3. Position the patient for a more detailed examination, in bed and undressed as far as is practical.
4. Watch for any difficulty the patient may have in undressing.

THE PRINCIPLES OF JOINT EXAMINATION

Look, **feel**, **move** and **measure** when examining the affected joints.

1. Look (compare right with left) for:
   - **Erythema:** redness of overlying skin suggests active **arthritis** or **infection** of the joint.
   - **Atrophy:** wasting of skin and its appendages suggests the condition is chronic.
   - **Scars:** previous operations may have been performed on the joint or associated tendons (e.g. joint replacement or tendon repair).
   - **Rashes:** (1) psoriasis, a scaly, silvery rash on the extensor surfaces, is associated with a number of types of arthritis; (2) vasculitis, which is inflammation of small arteries, causes skin (e.g. palpable purpura) and nail bed changes (e.g. linear haemorrhages) and can be associated with active arthritis (e.g. rheumatoid arthritis).
   - **Swelling** over the joint: this may be due to effusion (fluid accumulation within the joint space), hypertrophy or inflammation of the synovium (boggy swelling), or bony overgrowths at the joint margins (hard swelling in osteoarthritis).
   - **Deformity:** destructive arthritis causes distortion of the architecture of the area involved (e.g. the deviation of

the fingers towards the ulnar side of the hand in severe rheumatoid arthritis).

- **Subluxation:** displaced parts of the joint surfaces remain partly in contact.
- **Dislocation:** loss of contact between the joint surfaces occurs as a result of damage to the joint surfaces and the surrounding tissues and tendons.
- **Muscle wasting:** disuse, inflammation and sometimes nerve entrapment can all be responsible for the wasting of muscles near affected joints.

2. Feel for:
   - **Warmth:** active synovitis, infection or crystal arthritis (e.g. gout) all cause increased vascularity and make the area around the affected joint warmer than normal.
   - **Tenderness:** joint inflammation or infection is a likely cause.
   - **Synovitis:** this causes a very characteristic boggy swelling that is firmer than an effusion.
   - **Bony swelling:** osteophyte formation in osteoarthritis or subchondral bone thickening is very hard.

3. Move:
   - **Passive** movement: ask the patient to relax and let you move the joint in its normal anatomical directions; note limited extension (called **fixed flexion deformity**) or limited flexion (called **fixed extension deformity**).
   - **Active** movement: to assess integrated joint function (e.g. hand function, gait, neck and back examination), ask the patient to move the joint.
   - **Stability:** attempt to move the joint gently in abnormal directions; an unstable joint can be moved in directions other than its usual planes of movement because of dislocation or loss of normal tendon support.
   - **Joint crepitus:** place your hand over the joint or tendons as the patient moves the joint—a grating sensation or noise from the joint suggests chronicity.

4. Measure:
   - **Estimate** the approximate joint angles if indicated. Only rheumatologists can remember the joint angles in clinical practice but they are included for completeness.

Record movement as the number of degrees of flexion from the anatomical position in extension (e.g. straight knee). A knee with a fixed flexion deformity may be recorded as 30° to 60°, which indicates that there is 30° of fixed flexion deformity and that flexion is limited to 60°.

- **Use a tape measure** (1) to measure and follow serially the quadriceps muscle bulk and (2) in examination of spinal movements (see below).

EXAMINATION OF INDIVIDUAL JOINTS

You must know how to fully examine the hands, back and knees, although other joints can also provide important diagnostic information.

The hands and wrists

Sit the patient over the side of the bed and place the patient's hands on the pillow with the palms down.

1. Look:
   - **Wrists:** note erythema, atrophy, scars, swelling and rashes; also look for hollow ridges between the metacarpal bones (muscle wasting of the intrinsic muscles of the hand).
   - **Metacarpophalangeal joints:** note skin abnormalities, swelling or deformity (ulnar deviation and volar [palmar] subluxation of the fingers).
   - **Proximal interphalangeal** and **distal interphalangeal joints:** note skin changes and joint swelling.
   - **Swan neck deformity:** note flexion of proximal interphalangeal joints and hyperextension of distal interphalangeal joints—this is characteristic of rheumatoid arthritis (see Fig 11.3).
   - **Osteoarthritis:** note the presence of **swollen** distal interphalangeal and first carpometacarpal joints. Look for **Heberden's nodes**, which are marginal osteophytes that lie at the base of the distal phalanges.
   - **Fingers:** note the presence of the **typical sausage-shaped fingers** of psoriatic arthropathy.
   - **Nails:** note **psoriatic** nail changes such as pitting (see Table 3.2), onycholysis, hyperkeratosis (thickened nails), ridging and discolouration.

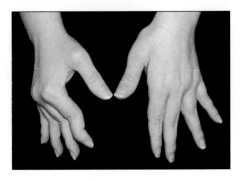

Figure 11.3 Swan neck deformity. (Sebastin SJ, Chung KC. Reconstruction of digital deformities in rheumatoid arthritis. *Hand Clinics* 2011; 27(1), Figure 4.)

- **Vasculitic** changes: look for linear haemorrhages (e.g. due to rheumatoid arthritis).
- **Palmar surfaces**: note scars (from tendon repairs or transfers), palmar erythema and muscle wasting of the thenar or hypothenar eminences.

2. Feel and move (see Fig 11.4):
   - Feel with your two thumbs at the **wrists** for **synovitis** (see Fig 11.5) and effusions. Note tenderness, limitation of movement or joint crepitus.
   - Go on to the metacarpophalangeal joints. **Flex the metacarpophalangeal joint** with the proximal phalanx held between the thumb and forefinger, then rock the joint backwards and forwards. Considerable movement may be present when ligamentous laxity or subluxation is present.
   - **Palpate all the proximal and distal interphalangeal joints** for tenderness and swelling. Bony swelling is hard and due to the presence of osteophytes.
   - Test for **palmar tendon crepitus**. Place the palmar aspects of your fingers against the palm of the patient's hand while he or she flexes and extends the metacarpophalangeal joints. Look for a **trigger finger** (inability to extend a finger in stenosing tenosynovitis).
   - Perform **Finkelstein's test**. Hold the patient's hand with the thumb tucked into the palm and then turn the wrist

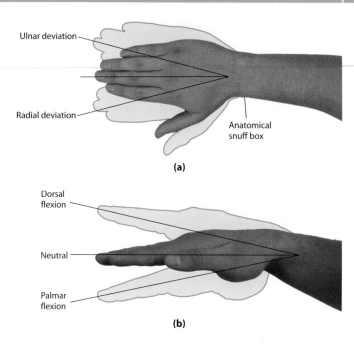

Figure 11.4 Movements of the wrist joint. **(a)** Ulnar and radial deviation. **(b)** Dorsal and palmar flexion. (Courtesy of Glenn McCulloch.)

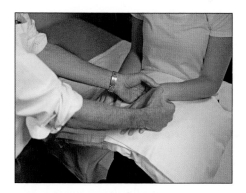

Figure 11.5 Feeling for synovitis at the wrists.

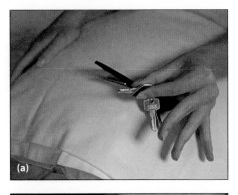

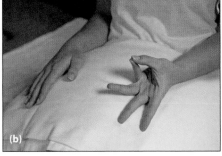

Figure 11.6   The key grip **(a)** and testing opposition strength **(b)**.

quickly into full ulnar deviation. Sharp pain will occur in the thumb tendons when there is tenosynovitis of these tendons (de Quervain's tenosynovitis).

- Feel for the **subcutaneous nodules** of rheumatoid arthritis near the elbows.

3. Test for function:

- Test for **grip strength** by getting the patient to squeeze two of your fingers.
- Test for **key grip** (see Fig 11.6a) by getting the patient to hold a key between the pulps of the thumb and forefinger.
- Test for **opposition strength** (see Fig 11.6b) by asking the patient to oppose the thumb and little finger, then assess the difficulty with which these can be forced apart.
- Perform a **practical test**, such as asking the patient to undo a button or write with a pen.

The elbows

1. Look for a **joint effusion** (a swelling on either side of the olecranon). Discrete swellings over the olecranon may be due to rheumatoid nodules (firm swellings that may be tender and are attached to deeper structures), gouty tophi or an enlarged olecranon bursa.
2. Feel for **tenderness**, particularly over the epicondyles. **Rheumatoid nodules** are hard, may be tender and are attached to underlying structures, whereas **gouty tophi** have a firm feeling and often appear yellow-coloured under the skin.
3. Move the elbow joints passively. The elbow is a hinge joint with movement from 0° (**extension**) to 150° (**flexion**).

The shoulders

1. Look at the joint (see Fig 11.7). Only large effusions can be detected.
2. Feel for tenderness and swelling.
3. Perform the Apley scratch test to examine active shoulder movement. Ask the patient to scratch an imaginary itch over the opposite scapula, first by reaching over the opposite shoulder, then by reaching behind the neck and then by reaching behind the back (see Fig 11.8). Look for restricted movement and ask about pain during the various movements.
4. If the scratch test is abnormal, move the joint passively. Test **abduction** (90°), **elevation** (180°), **adduction** (50°), **external rotation** (60°), **internal rotation** (90°), **flexion** (180°) and **extension** (65°) (see Fig 11.7). Watch to make sure movement is of the shoulder and not of the scapula.

The temporomandibular joints

1. Look in front of the ear for swelling.
2. Feel for grating and tenderness by placing a finger just in front of the ear while the patient opens and shuts the mouth.

The neck

1. Look at the cervical spine while the patient is sitting up and note particularly the patient's posture.
2. Test **movement** actively for **flexion** (45°), **extension** (45°), **lateral bending** (45°) and **rotation** (70°) (see Fig 11.9).

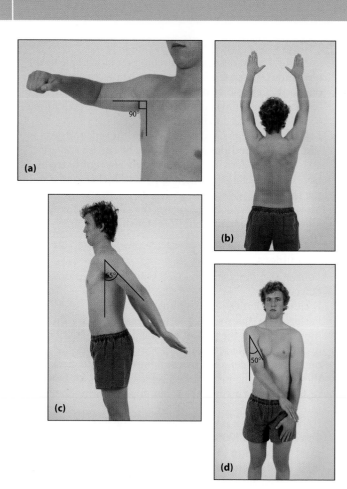

Figure 11.7 Movements of the shoulders. **(a)** Abduction using the glenohumeral joint. **(b)** Abduction using the glenohumeral joint and the scapula. **(c)** Extension. **(d)** Adduction. (Courtesy of Glenn McCulloch.)

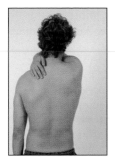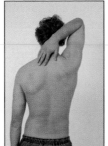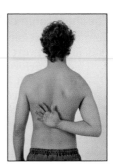

Figure 11.8   Apley scratch test to assess shoulder movement. (Courtesy of Glenn McCulloch.)

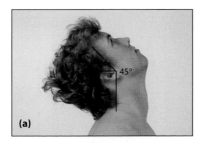

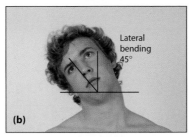

Figure 11.9   Movements of the neck. **(a)** Extension—'Look up and back.' **(b)** Lateral bending—'Now touch your right ear onto your shoulder' (45°). Rotation—'Now look over your shoulder to the right and then to the left' (70°). (Courtesy of Glenn McCulloch.)

The thoracolumbar spine and sacroiliac joints

To start the examination, have the patient standing and clothed only in underwear.

1. Look for **deformity** such as scoliosis, a lateral curvature of the spine or loss of the normal thoracic kyphosis, and lumbar lordosis (e.g. due to ankylosing spondylitis).
2. Feel **each vertebral body** for tenderness and palpate for muscle spasm. Also feel for sacroiliac joint tenderness.
3. Test movement actively: **flexion, extension, lateral bending** and **rotation** (see Fig 11.10). Measure the extent

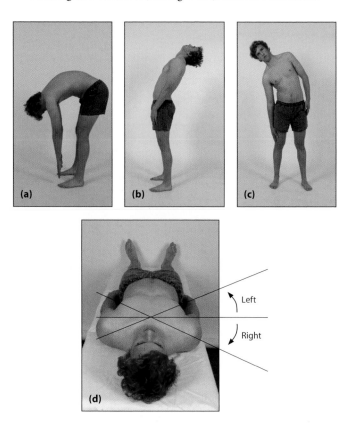

Figure 11.10 Movements of the thoracolumbar spine. **(a)** Flexion. **(b)** Extension. **(c)** Lateral bending. **(d)** Rotation. (Courtesy of Glenn McCulloch.)

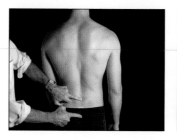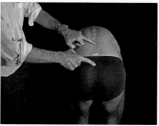

Figure 11.11 Schober's test.

of lumbar flexion using Schober's test (see Fig 11.11). Make a mark at the level of the posterior iliac spine on the vertebral column. Place one finger 5 cm below this mark and one finger 10 cm above. Ask the patient to bend and touch his or her toes. If lumbar flexion is normal, the distance between your fingers should increase by at least 5 cm.

4. Assess **straight leg raising**, with the patient lying down, by lifting the straightened leg. In lumbar disc prolapse (L4, L5, S1 nerve roots) this will be limited by pain.

5. Perform the **femoral nerve stretch test**. Ask the patient to lie on his or her front (prone). Flex the knee then extend the hip. Pain in the back (or front of the thigh) is a positive test.

The hips

1. Feel just distal to the midpoint of the inguinal ligament for joint tenderness.

2. Move the hip joint passively with the patient lying down, first on the back.

3. Test **flexion** (90°), **abduction** (50°), **adduction** (45°) **external rotation** and **internal rotation** (45°). Ask the patient to roll over onto the stomach and test **extension** (see Fig 11.12).

4. Ask the patient to stand and perform the **Trendelenburg test**. The patient stands first on one leg and then on the other. Normally the non-weightbearing hip rises, but with proximal myopathy or hip joint disease the non-weightbearing side sags.

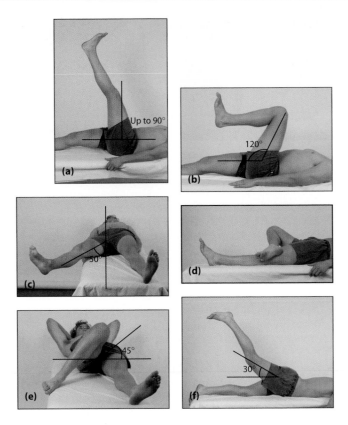

Figure 11.12 Movements of the hip. **(a)** Flexion. **(b)** Flexion, knee bent. **(c)** Abduction. **(d)** External rotation. **(e)** Internal rotation. **(f)** Extension. (Courtesy of Glenn McCulloch.)

The knees

1. Look for quadriceps wasting and examine the knees themselves for skin changes, swelling and deformity. A space will be visible under the knee if there is a permanent flexion deformity. The knee then cannot be extended fully and remains permanently flexed so that it cannot lie flat on the bed.

2. Feel the quadriceps for **wasting**. Palpate over the knees for warmth and synovial swelling.

3. Use the **patellar tap** to confirm the presence of large effusions. Compress the lower end of the quadriceps muscle and push any fluid contained in the suprapatellar bursa down and under the patella. Use your other hand to push down briskly on the patella. The presence of posterior displacement of the patella followed by a palpable and audible tap is a sign of a significant fluid collection. Smaller amounts of fluid may be indicated by a fullness on either side of the patella; with milking movements upwards the fluid may be seen temporarily to diminish and then slowly accumulate.

4. Move the joint passively. Test **flexion** (135°) and **extension** (5°), and note the presence of crepitus (see Fig 11.13a).

5. Test the **collateral** and **cruciate ligaments**. The lateral and medial collateral ligaments are tested by having the patient flex the knee slightly. Rest your arm along the patient's tibia

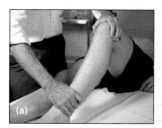
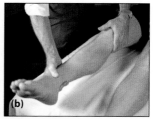
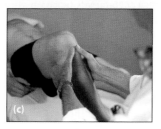

Figure 11.13   Examining the knee joints. **(a)** Testing for crepitus. **(b)** Testing the collateral ligaments. **(c)** Testing the cruciate ligaments.

and attempt lateral and medial movements of the leg on the knee. The thigh is steadied with your other hand (see Fig 11.13b). Movement of more than 10° is abnormal. The cruciate ligaments are tested by flexing the patient's knee to 90°. One hand steadies the thigh while the other, placed behind the patient's knee, attempts to produce anterior and posterior movements of the leg on the knee joint (see Fig 11.13c).

6. Finally, stand the patient up. Look particularly for **varus** (bow leg) and **valgus** (knock-knee) deformity.

7. Look and feel behind the knees in the **popliteal fossa** for a Baker's cyst.

The ankles and feet

1. Look at the skin for swelling, deformity (hallux valgus and clawing) or muscle wasting. **Sausage-like deformities of the toes** occur with psoriatic arthropathy, ankylosing spondylitis and Reiter's disease. Look for the nail changes that suggest psoriasis. Inspect the transverse arch of the foot and the longitudinal arch; these may be flattened in arthritic conditions of the foot.

2. Feel for **swelling** around the lateral and medial malleoli. Painless swelling and disorganisation of the ankle occur with a Charcot's joint—often due to a diabetic neuropathy.

3. Move the **talar (ankle) joint**, grasping the mid-foot with one hand (**dorsiflexion** and **plantar flexion**).

4. With the **subtalar joint**, tenderness on movement is more important than range of movement.

5. Squeeze the **metatarsophalangeal joints** by compressing the first and fifth metatarsals between your thumb and forefinger. Tenderness suggests inflammation.

6. Palpate the **Achilles tendon** for rheumatoid nodules or Achilles tendonitis.

T&O'C examination essentials

Common rheumatological abnormalities
Hands
Rheumatoid arthritis (see Figs 11.3 and 11.14)
Osteoarthritis
Gouty arthritis
Psoriatic arthritis and nails
Scleroderma

Back
Ankylosing spondylitis

Knees
Osteoarthritis
Effusion

Ankles and feet
Rheumatoid arthritis of the feet
Charcot's joint ankle
Gout

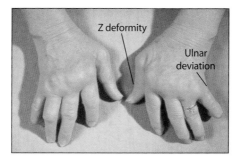

Figure 11.14 Rheumatoid arthritis hands with arrows pointing to typical deformities. (Sebastin SJ, Chung KC. Reconstruction of digital deformities in rheumatoid arthritis. *Hand Clinics* 2011; 27(1), Figure 4.)

T&O'C examination essentials

How to assess a patient's rheumatological system, including mobility, quickly

Use a modified **GALS** method:
Gait
Arms
Legs
Spine.

Ask
1. Are you troubled by pain or stiffness in your back, muscles or joints?
2. Where?
3. How are you affected by this?
4. Can you walk up and down stairs?
5. Can you get out of a chair easily?
6. Can you wash and dress yourself?

Examine
1. **Gait.** Ask the patient to walk to the end of the room, turn around and come back. Note the length of stride, smoothness of walking and turning around, stance, heel strike and arm swing. Is walking obviously painful or is there a neurological problem? A Parkinsonian gait, foot drop or other neurological gait should be obvious.
2. **Arms, legs and spine.**
   (a) **From behind:** look at the spine for scoliosis. Is the muscle bulk of the shoulders, paraspinal muscles, gluteal muscles and calves symmetrical and normal?
   (b) **From the side:** look for normal lordosis and thoracic kyphosis. Ask the patient to bend and look for normal separation of the lumbar spinous processes.
   (c) **From in front:** look for asymmetry or wasting of major muscle groups (shoulders, arms and quadriceps). Is there any deformity of the knees, ankles or feet?
3. When arthritis seems to be an important part of the case, take the time to test movement. Look for restricted, asymmetrical or painful movements.
   (a) **Spine.**
      • Rotation: 'Turn your shoulders as far as you can to the right; now to the left.'
      • Lateral flexion: 'Slide your hand down the side of your leg on the right side; repeat on the left.'
      • Cervical spine:
         – Lateral flexion: 'Bend your right ear down towards your right shoulder; repeat on the left.'
         – Flexion and extension: 'Look up and back as far as you can; now put your chin on your chest.'

T&O'C examination essentials *continued*

(b) **Shoulders** (acromioclavicular, glenohumeral, sternoclavicular joints).
- 'Put your right hand on your back and reach up as far as you can as if to scratch your back; repeat with your left hand.'
- 'Put your hands up behind your head and your elbows as far back as you can.'

(c) **Elbows (extension).**
- 'With your elbows straight, put your arms down beside you.'

(d) **Hands and wrists.**
- 'Straighten out your arms and hands in front of you.'
  - Look for fixed flexion deformity of the fingers and swelling and deformity of the hands and wrists or wasting of the small muscles of the hands.
- 'Turn your hands up the other way.'
  - Look at the palms for swelling or muscle wasting.
  - Is supination smooth and complete?
  - Is external rotation of the shoulder used to make up for limited supination?
- 'Squeeze my fingers as hard as you can.' (Tests for grip strength.)
- 'Touch the tip of each finger with your thumb.' (Tests most finger joints.)

(e) **Legs and hips.**
- 'Lie down on the bed for me.'
  - Look at leg length and, if suspicious, measure true leg length from the anterior superior iliac spine to the medial malleolus and apparent length from the umbilicus to the medial malleolus.
  - Test knee flexion.
- 'Bend your knee and pull your foot up towards your bottom.'
  - Put your hand on the patella and feel for crepitus.
- Test for osteoarthritis of the hip by internally rotating the hip.
- Flex the knee to 90° and move the foot laterally.
- Pain and limitation of movement occur early with osteoarthritis.

(f) **Feet.**
- Look for arthritic changes, especially at the metatarsophalangeal joints, bunions, calluses etc.

The examination will have to be varied for very immobile patients, but with practice it can be performed rapidly and should easily satisfy your examiners.

The joints OSCE: hints panel

1. This woman has rheumatoid arthritis. Please take a history from her to assess the severity of the disease and its effect on her.
   (a) Ask her the following:
      (i) How old are you? How old were you when your joint problems began?
      (ii) What joints have been involved and at roughly what times?
      (iii) Do you currently have any active arthritis (morning stiffness, any swelling)? For how long? What joints? Is it worse with exercise or rest?
      (iv) What has been and is your occupation? How do you cope at work? Do you feel confident about continuing to work?
      (v) Can you drive? How do you manage bathing, dressing, toileting, etc?
      (vi) Who lives at home with you? How do these people cope with your illness?
      (vii) Has your house or car had to be modified? Do you need a walking stick, frame or wheelchair?
      (viii) What treatment are you on? Have you required steroids? Have the drugs caused any problems? Have you required treatment for osteoporosis or anaemia?
      (ix) Have you had joint or tendon surgery?
      (x) Are you concerned about your future health?
   (b) Synthesise and present your findings.
2. This man has painful hands. Please examine them. (Wash your hands)
   (a) Stand back to look at the patient for obvious generalised arthritis.
   (b) Ask him to sit up in a chair or with his legs over the edge of the bed and rest his hands on a pillow.
   (c) Look at the palmar and dorsal surfaces before touching his hands. Note any deformities.
   (d) Ask whether there are any areas of tenderness.
   (e) Examine his hands as outlined on p. 264.
   (f) Present your findings at the end, or describe any abnormalities as you go along.
3. This patient has right knee pain on walking. Please examine him. (Wash your hands)
   (a) Ask the patient to expose both of his legs to at least the mid-thigh.
   (b) Test gait. Look from the front and the sides.
   (c) While the patient gets back on the bed, stand back and look for more general abnormalities, including deformities of other major joints.
   (d) Now inspect his knees. Look for obvious signs of inflammation or deformity. Is there an obvious effusion?

   (e) Ask whether his knees are tender. Feel his knees. Note any tenderness and the skin temperature. Note any effusion.
   (f) Assess knee movements, crepitus and ligament stability.
   (g) Synthesise and present your findings.
4. This man has had lower back pain. Please examine his back. (Wash your hands)
   (a) Ask the patient to undress to his underpants.
   (b) Watch him undressing for problems with immobility or pain.
   (c) Look at his back for deformity (increased or reduced thoracic kyphosis or lumbar lordosis, scoliosis) and for scars from previous back surgery.
   (d) Ask about tenderness. Palpate each vertebral body and the sacroiliac joints. Use your closed fist to gently percuss for tenderness.
   (e) Test the range of movement, asking whether movement is painful each time ('touch your toes with straight legs', 'lean back as far as possible', 'reach down to the side and touch below your knee').
   (f) Ask the patient to lie in bed and perform straight leg raising and the femoral nerve stretch test.
   (g) Synthesise and present your findings.
5. Please assess this woman's hand function. (Wash your hands)
   (a) Look at her hands for deformity and swelling.
   (b) Ask whether they are tender.
   (c) Ask her to perform various tasks to test hand function: key grip (opposition and adduction of thumb), pinch grip (opposition and flexion of thumb) and dressing (hand, elbow, shoulder).
   (d) Ask to perform a neurological examination of her hand for peripheral nerve or sensory lesions.
   (e) Synthesise and present your findings.

T&O'C examination essentials

Examination of the joints
1. Ask about pain and stiffness in all the joints.
2. Determine the actual joint involvement by history and confirm this on examination.
3. Always compare an affected joint with the opposite joint to ascertain the amount of abnormality.
4. Inflamed joints are usually hot, red, swollen and tender. Impaired function is also present.
5. Functional assessment of involved joints gives important information about the clinical impact of a condition.
6. Distinguishing non-specific lower back pain from that of ankylosing spondylitis is difficult, but tenderness to pressure over the sacroiliac joints is a helpful sign of the latter.

The skin

*Half of us are blind, few of us feel, and we are
all deaf.*

Sir William Osler (1849–1919)

The dermatological history

You may have noticed a rash during the examination that the
patient forgot to mention (look not just with your eyes but with
your brain, then you will see) or the patient may have presented
because of a concern about a skin problem. In either case, certain
questions should be asked:

1. How long has the lesion or abnormality been present?
2. Has its distribution changed over time? Has it changed in
   colour or become irregular or bigger?
3. Has it been associated with sun exposure or exposure to
   heat or cold?
4. Is there associated pruritus (itch)? (Itch can be due to
   local skin disease [e.g. dry skin, atopic dermatitis, scabies]
   or a systemic disease [e.g. obstructive jaundice, chronic
   renal failure, lymphoma])
5. Is the lesion painful or associated with altered sensation?
6. Does the patient have constitutional symptoms (fever, loss
   of weight, headache etc)?
7. Does the patient have a past history of skin disease or
   atopy (allergy)?

8. Does the patient have a history of systemic disease (e.g. inflammatory bowel disease, diabetes mellitus, connective tissue disease, arthritis)?
9. Does the patient have a history of exposure to chemicals, animals or plants?
10. Does the patient have a family history of melanoma? (10% of melanomas are associated with a history of the disease in first-degree relatives)
11. What medications is the patient taking?

Examination anatomy

Figure 12.1 shows the three main layers of the skin:

- epidermis
- dermis
- subcutaneous fat.

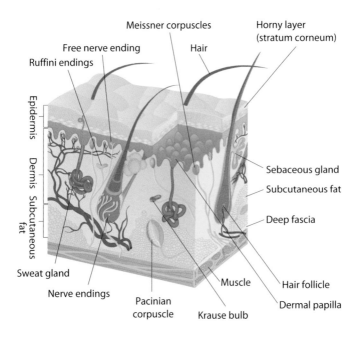

Figure 12.1 The three main layers of the skin.

These layers can all be involved in skin diseases in varying combinations. Most skin tumours arise in the epidermis. Skin appendages such as hair follicles (see Fig 12.2) are a common site of infection, especially in adolescents and people on steroid medications (acne).

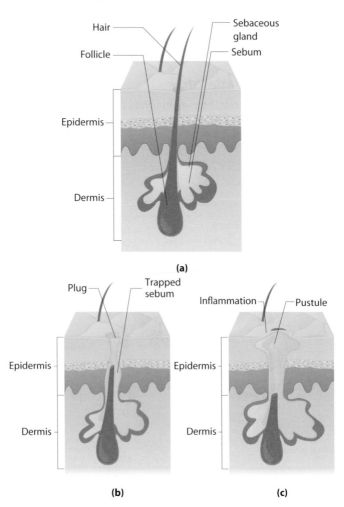

Figure 12.2 **(a)** Clear skin. **(b)** Blackhead. **(c)** Infected follicle.

Examination of the skin

Look actively and systematically at all areas of the skin. Craft your own system (e.g. front then back; start at the face and proceed down) to cover the entire skin surface. The patient should undress so that the whole surface of the skin is accessible.

1. **Describe** any lesions according to their colour, size and shape and using dermatological terms (see Table 12.1).
2. Note their **distribution**.
3. Describe the **pattern** (see Table 12.2).
4. **Palpate** the lesions, noting the consistency, tenderness, temperature, depth within the skin and mobility of any lesion and the skin overlying it.

TABLE 12.1	Dermatological terms
Atrophy	Thinning of the epidermis with loss of normal skin markings
Bulla	A large collection of fluid below the epidermis
Crust	Dried serum and exudate
Ecchymoses	Bruises
Excoriations	Lesions caused by scratching that results in loss of the epidermis
Keloid	Hypertrophic scarring
Macule	A circumscribed alteration of skin colour
Nodule	A circumscribed palpable mass greater than 1 cm in diameter
Papule	A circumscribed palpable elevation less than 1 cm in diameter

continued

TABLE 12.1 Dermatological terms *continued*	
Petechiae	Red, non-blanching spots <5 mm
Pigment alterations	Increased (hyperpigmentation) or decreased (hypopigmentation)
Plaque	A palpable, disc-shaped lesion
Purpura	Red, non-blanching spots >5 mm
Pustule	A visible collection of pus
Scales	An accumulation of excess keratin
Sclerosis	Induration of subcutaneous tissues that may involve the dermis
Ulcer	A circumscribed loss of tissue
Vesicle	A small collection of fluid below the epidermis
Wheal	An area of dermal oedema

TABLE 12.2 Patterns in dermatology	
Annular	Ring-shaped (hollow centre) (e.g. tinea infection)
Arcuate	Curved (e.g. secondary syphilis)
Circinate	Circular
Confluent	Lesions that have run together (e.g. measles)
Discoid	Circular without a hollow centre (e.g. lupus)
Eczematous	Inflamed and crusted (e.g. allergic eczema)
Keratotic	Thickened from increased keratin (e.g. psoriasis)
Lichenified	Thickening and roughening of the epidermis associated with accentuated skin markings
Linear	In lines (e.g. contact dermatitis)
Nodular	Raised solid lesion >10 mm (e.g. erythema nodosum)
Papular	Raised solid lesion <10 mm (e.g. wart)
Papulosquamous	Plaques associated with scaling
Reticulated	In a network pattern (e.g. cutaneous parasite)
Serpiginous	Sinuous
Zosteriform	Following a nerve distribution (e.g. herpes zoster)

SKIN TUMOURS

Skin tumours are very common skin lesions. Most are benign, but malignant tumours must be recognised early (see Box 12.1 and Figs 12.3 and 12.4), because successful treatment depends on early diagnosis. Primary skin cancers of all types are more common in people with fair skin who have been exposed to the sun. Many cancers will eventually ulcerate as they outgrow their blood supply. All non-healing ulcers should be considered malignant until proved benign.

- **Solar keratoses** are premalignant. They may begin as pink macules often surrounded by adherent scale. They often feel rough, like sandpaper. A proportion of them regress spontaneously.
- **Basal cell carcinomas** begin as a papule with a depressed centre and have a rolled border that has a characteristic pearly appearance (see Fig 12.3b).
- **Squamous cell carcinomas** begin as an opaque papule or plaque that is often eroded or scaly (see Fig 12.3a).
- **Malignant melanomas** often appear as deeply pigmented lesions with an irregular border (see Fig 12.3c). They enlarge and often develop patchy changes in pigment colour. They tend to be asymmetrical.

Remember to note the features on the ABCD checklist (see Box 12.2).

Box 12.1
Skin tumours

- Solar keratoses (actinic)—premalignant
- Basal cell carcinoma
- Squamous cell carcinoma
- Bowen's disease (squamous cell carcinoma confined to the epithelial layer of the skin—carcinoma in situ)
- Malignant melanoma
- Secondary deposits

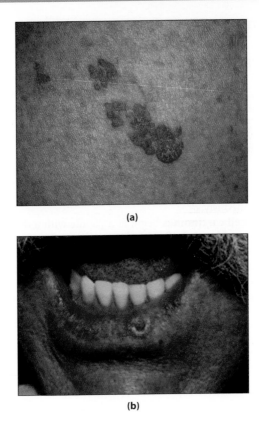

(a)

(b)

Figure 12.3   **(a)** Squamous cell carcinoma, in situ, Bowen's type. Scaly red plaque on the chest with skip areas. (Bolognia JL et al. *Dermatology Essential*. Elsevier; 2014, Fig. 88.3.) **(b)** Basal cell carcinoma. The lower lip is a relatively commonly affected site. (White GM, Cox NH [eds]. *Diseases of the Skin: A Color Atlas and Text 2e*. St Louis: Mosby; 2006.)

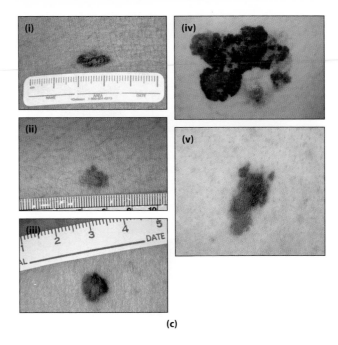

(c)

Figure 12.3, continued   **(c)** Superficial spreading melanomas.
(i)–(iii) All of these early lesions demonstrate asymmetry due to
variations in colour and irregularity in outline. In addition, there is pink
discolouration in (iii). (i) and (ii) were less than 0.5 mm in thickness and
(iii) was 0.8 mm. **(iv)** In this more advanced lesion, note the asymmetry,
irregular borders, variation in colour, scarlike regression zones and an
inferior pink papule, indicating vertical growth phase. **(v)** A superficial
spreading melanoma arising within a compound melanocytic nevus.
Note the irregular outline and variable pigmentation. ((i) Courtesy Kalman
Watsky. (ii), (iii), Courtesy Jean L. Bolognia. (iv) Courtesy Claus Garbe in
Bolognia JL et al. *Dermatology Essentials*. Elsevier; 2014, Fig. 93.5.)

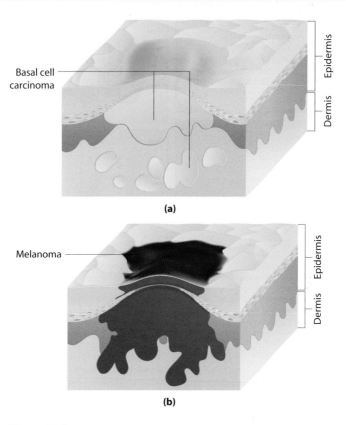

Figure 12.4 **(a)** Basal cell carcinoma. **(b)** Melanoma.

Box 12.2
Melanomas (ABCD checklist)[1]

Are typically **A**symmetrical
Have an irregular **B**order
Have an irregular **C**olour
Can be large in **D**iameter

---

1 Often asked for in an exam.

WOUNDS

Inspect any wounds and then, if appropriate, palpate them carefully while wearing gloves. Note:

- appearance
- exact site
- orientation (e.g. vertical or horizontal, localised or penetrating).

Determine whether a wound is just a bruise (bleeding under the skin), an abrasion (loss of just outer skin) or a scratch (linear abrasion), or more seriously a sharp or blunt (ragged edges) laceration, or most seriously a penetrating deep wound.

The skin OSCE: hints panel

This man has a pigmented lesion on his chest. Please assess him.
(a) Ask him the following:
  (i) Did you have much sun exposure in childhood?
  (ii) Do you have a family history of melanoma?
  (iii) When did you first notice the lesion? Is it new?
  (iv) Has the lesion changed in appearance?
  (v) Do you have any itching or bleeding?
  (vi) Have you had this lesion, or any other pigmented lesion, biopsied or excised?
(b) Inspect the lesion. Note whether it is symmetrical or not, has a regular or irregular border, is raised or not and has uniform or variable pigmentation, and look for any ulceration or inflammation. Measure the lesion's size. Consider making a photographic record for later comparison.
(c) Inspect the skin all over his body, including in his hair, for other pigmented lesions.
(d) Note the features on the ABCD checklist (melanomas are typically asymmetrical, have an irregular border, have an irregular colour and can be large in diameter).
(e) If this could be a melanoma, request a surgical biopsy.
(f) Synthesise and present your findings.

Assessment of the geriatric patient

Age is an issue of mind over matter. If you don't mind, it doesn't matter.

Samuel Clemens *(Mark Twain)* (1835–1910)

Generally defined as individuals aged 65 years or older, geriatric patients tend to report fewer symptoms but have more numerous chronic diseases. Disease presentation is more likely to be atypical, so spending time taking the history is critical. Patients may have hearing loss, difficulty seeing and cognitive impairment, which can all impair history taking.

History taking in the geriatric patient: special considerations

1. **Presenting symptoms:** these are usually multiple.
2. **Past history:** the immunisation status, especially for pneumococcus, influenza, tetanus and varicella zoster, should be recorded.
3. **Medications:** many patients will be taking multiple medications for several diseases, not all of which they may really need (polypharmacy). A comprehensive list, including reason for use, is important in terms of planning management.

4. **Social history:**
   - **Smoking habits:** details should be acquired as usual. Stopping smoking improves lung function, even in patients over the age of 60. Furthermore, advice to stop smoking is as successful in older patients as it is in younger ones.
   - **Exercise:** exercise is generally safe in the elderly and improves flexibility, balance, endurance and strength, which can assist with maintenance of independent function as well as improving quality of life.
   - **Living arrangements:** ask whether there is someone to help the patient in the home, if required.
   - **Vulnerability:** abuse and neglect can be problems in this age group. Try to find out whether the patient feels under threat from anyone.
5. **Systems review:**
   - Focus especially on vision, hearing, chewing and dentition, weight change, stool and urinary incontinence, recurrent falls, a history of fractures and foot disease.
   - Find out whether the patient has had a problem with falls, and particularly if any injuries have occurred. Falls are an important cause of mortality in the elderly and are usually multi-factorial: postural dizziness, poor vision, cognitive impairment, foot problems and gait problems can all contribute to or exacerbate the problem. A history of falls means that careful enquiry must be made about these associated factors. Impaired bone mineral density means a fracture is more likely to result from a fall.
   - Ask about symptoms of depression, because this is a common problem in the elderly and needs to be recognised and treated.
6. **Specific areas of enquiry:**
   - **Physical activities of daily living (ADLs):** ask the patient how he or she copes with bathing, dressing, toileting and handling money—these can be affected by many different chronic illnesses.
   - **Instrumental activities of daily living (IADLs):** ask the patient whether he or she has any difficulty using the

telephone, shopping, preparing food, housekeeping, doing the laundry, driving and taking medicines.

- **End-of-life and treatment decisions:** patients generally prefer their clinician to actively bring up this topic. It is worth encouraging the patient to write down his or her preferences about such decisions—for example, 'Do not resuscitate' orders.

Mental state examination

Any patient who has a history of confusion, or is suspected of having dementia or a major psychiatric illness, should undergo a mental state examination. Test for orientation, memory and attention. Even gross disturbances of these functions may not be obvious unless they are formally tested.

A simple screening tool for cognitive impairment is the Mini Cog™ test (3 steps, 3 minutes):

1. Ask the patient to remember 3 words (and repeat these up to 3 times to ensure that they have been captured by the patient).
2. Ask the patient to draw a clock face with all the numbers and then add the hands at a specific time (e.g. 10 minutes past 11 o'clock).
3. Ask the patient to repeat the 3 original words.

Scoring is out of 5: score 1 point for each correct word and 2 points for a fully correct clock face (0 if not fully correct). A total score of 0–2 suggests that formal testing for dementia is indicated.

An alternative approach is the Abbreviated Mental Test (AMT). Ask the patient the following:

1. State your age
2. State your date of birth
3. Give the current time (to the nearest hour)
4. Give the year
5. Give the hospital name
6. Identify two people (e.g. doctors)
7. Recall an address
8. State the dates of World War II (or another important event)
9. Name the Prime Minister or President (or equivalent)
10. Count backwards from 20 to 1

Score 1 point for each correct answer. A score of ≤8 out of 10 is abnormal.

The physical examination in the geriatric patient: special considerations

A complete examination is required as usual, but consider the following areas as you go about obtaining the data.

1. **General assessment:**
   - Check for postural blood pressure change.
   - Assess hydration, which may be impaired in older patients with cognitive dysfunction.
   - Look at the skin carefully for pressure sores or evidence of bruises from falls or elder abuse. Look at the skin for any evidence of skin cancer.
   - Measure the patient's weight and height to calculate the body mass index, as weight loss is common in the elderly.

2. **Heart:**
   - If a systolic murmur is heard, consider whether this may be aortic stenosis, which, if severe, is likely to require treatment.
   - Ankle swelling may indicate venous insufficiency or antihypertensive drug use (e.g. calcium antagonists) rather than congestive cardiac failure. Ischaemic heart disease is common but often silent in the elderly.

3. **Chest:**
   - Shortness of breath may be due to lung disease or cardiac disease, and these often coexist in the elderly.

4. **Gastrointestinal system:**
   - Look at the dentition and check for dry mouth, which may impair eating.
   - The abdominal aorta may be palpable in the thin elderly patient. This may be falsely interpreted as an aneurysm, but if the aorta seems significantly enlarged, an aortic aneurysm needs to be excluded. If the aneurysm is leaking, the classical presentation includes back pain, abdominal distension, shock and poor asymmetrical peripheral pulses in the legs.

- In patients with constipation from hard stool, a mass may be felt in the left lower quadrant: this will clear with treatment for the constipation.
- Perform a rectal examination and rule out faecal impaction, particularly if there is a history of faecal or urinary incontinence.
- In patients with acute urinary retention, an enlarged bladder may be felt: this problem can present with delirium.

5. **Nervous system:**
   - Evaluation of mental status should be routine in geriatric patients.
   - Check for the following primitive reflexes which are found in the elderly and may be evidence of dementia: glabellar tap (tap with your fingertip between the eyebrows—if abnormal, blinking continues after 3–4 taps), snout (tap the lips—lip protrusion is abnormal), palmar mental reflex (stroke with the tongue depressor from the thenar eminence to the base of the thumb and look at the chin—if abnormal, the chin will wrinkle) and grasp reflex (stroke the palm firmly with your finger, beginning on the radial side—if your finger is gripped it is abnormal).
   - Test gait with the 'get up and go' test. Ask the patient to stand up from a chair, walk 3 metres, turn around 180°, return to the chair and sit down.

6. **Eyes and ears:**
   - Check vision and hearing as these may impair independent living.

7. **Rheumatological system:**
   - Examine for deformities and functional disabilities, including the feet.

8. **Breasts:**
   - Perform a breast examination in women, as the incidence of breast cancer greatly increases with age.

Assessment of the acutely ill patient

There is no disease more conducive to clinical humility than aneurysm of the aorta.

Sir William Osler (1849–1919)

During your training, you will be expected to become expert in basic cardiac life support and advanced cardiac life support, and this training must be refreshed regularly.

If you come across an obviously very ill patient, the first step is to ask: 'Are you all right?'

- If the patient is **unresponsive** on gentle shaking, check whether the airway is patent and whether he or she is breathing, and then assess the circulation.
  - Start cardiopulmonary resuscitation if the patient is not breathing or has no pulse, and try to send someone else to call for help.
  - Examine the patient for any evidence of obvious bleeding or other trauma: if he or she does not require resuscitation, proceed to a more detailed assessment.
- If the patient is clearly **responding appropriately** to questions, and has skin that is normal in colour as well as being warm and dry, he or she is much less likely to need urgent intervention before appropriate history taking and a targeted physical examination can be done.

- Gather key data as summarised by the mnemonic, AMPLE:

  Allergies
  Medication currently being taken and most recent medications taken
  Past medical history
  Last meal
  Events preceding the current incident.

- If the patient is **tachypnoeic**, check pulse oximetry and start oxygen therapy unless there is a known contraindication.
- If the patient is **bradycardic** or **tachycardic**, check the blood pressure and obtain an electrocardiogram (ECG).
- If the patient is **hypotensive**, consider an intravenous fluid challenge and measure the heart rate, blood pressure, respiratory rate and hourly urinary output (if necessary by placing a urinary catheter). Assess capillary refill time by depressing the patient's fingernail or toenail until it blanches and record the time it takes for the colour to become normal again; this is usually less than 2 seconds. A delayed capillary refill time occurs in hypovolaemic or cardiogenic shock.
- Examine the patient's chest for any obvious evidence of **tension pneumothorax** (characterised by dyspnoea, tachycardia, absent breath sounds over the side of the tension pneumothorax and tracheal deviation away from the affected side, and there may be jugular venous distension). Assess the patient for possible **cardiac tamponade** (which can present with distended neck veins as well as low blood pressure and pulsus paradoxus). Measure the patient's temperature. If this is elevated, consider taking blood and urine cultures (before beginning antibiotic treatment).
- If the patient's **level of consciousness becomes impaired** during your assessment, recheck the airway, breathing and circulation (ABCs), check the serum glucose (**you must not miss hypoglycaemia**) and obtain intravenous access immediately.

T&O'C examination hint box

ABC = **A**irway, **B**reathing, **C**irculation.

Remember, if the patient is in cardiac arrest (hint: the patient is unresponsive), your first job is to quickly initiate excellent cardiopulmonary resuscitation (CPR) focusing initially on the **C**irculation (rapid chest compressions), then the **A**irway, then **B**reathing (CAB, the new ABC). You must become proficient in basic and advanced cardiac life support.

Note: If a patient who is on a cardiac monitor is seen to go into ventricular fibrillation, the patient should have immediate DC cardioversion if this is available. Cardioversion should not be delayed so that CPR can be commenced.

Assess level of consciousness using the AVPU system:

Alert (normal)
Verbal stimulus responsive
Painful stimulus responsive
Unresponsive.

Formally assess the patient using the Glasgow Coma Scale (see Box 14.1). Record the results as the total score (e.g. GCS 10/15) and the three component scores (e.g. E3, M5, V2).

Box 14.1
The Glasgow Coma Scale

Add up the scores for 1, 2 and 3: a total score of 4 or less = very poor prognosis for recovery; a total score >11 = good prognosis for recovery.

1 Eyes	Open	Spontaneously	4
		To loud verbal command	3
		To pain	2
	No response		1
2 Best motor response	To verbal command	Obeys	6
		Localises pain	5
	To painful stimuli	Flexion—withdrawal	4
		Abnormal flexion posturing	3
		Extension posturing	2
	No response		1
3 Best verbal response		Oriented	5
		Confused, disoriented	4
		Inappropriate words	3
		Incomprehensible sounds	2
		None	1

This man has had episodes of sudden loss of consciousness. Please examine him.

(a) Assess his level of consciousness, response to commands or pain, and spontaneous movement of limbs.

(b) If he is not unconscious, test orientation to time, place and person.

(c) Examine his gait, then his limbs and cranial nerves, looking for focal neurological signs (stroke, intracranial tumour).

(d) Note whether there are tongue lacerations (seizures).

(e) Take his pulse (arrhythmias including atrial fibrillation or heart block), and blood pressure lying down and sitting (postural hypotension).

(f) Examine the praecordium (signs of new murmurs, tamponade).

(g) Take his temperature and assess for neck stiffness (sepsis, meningism).

(h) Check the blood sugar with a skin-prick test (especially if a diabetic).

(i) Synthesise and present your findings.

15

Examining the systems of the body

There is no more difficult art to acquire than the art of observation, and for some men[1] it is quite as difficult to record an observation in brief and plain language.

Sir William Osler (1849–1919)

This chapter summarises suggested approaches to examination of the major body systems. There is no single correct method, however, and you should develop one that suits you and ensures you leave nothing out.

In the hospital medical record, it is routine to record the major findings in the cardiovascular, respiratory, abdominal and neurological systems. Other systems (e.g. joints) are included based on the history. The presenting history should guide the detail sought in the relevant system examinations. In a short case examination or OSCE you will often be given an introduction to the patient's symptoms and asked to examine a system—for example, 'This man has noticed double vision. Please examine his cranial nerves.' Always step back and observe before starting your detailed assessments.

A complete assessment is as follows.

---

1 Women *and* men, of course, may suffer from this difficulty.

The cardiovascular system (see Fig 15.1)

1. Arrange for the patient to lie at 45° and make sure the patient's chest and neck are fully exposed. Cover the breasts of a female patient with a towel or loose garment. Stand on the right side of the bed.
2. Stand back and inspect for **dyspnoea**, **cyanosis** (central or peripheral blue discolouration of the mucous membranes

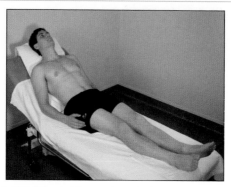

Lay the patient at 45° and make sure the patient's head and neck are fully exposed.

General inspection
Marfan's syndrome,
   Turner's syndrome,
   Down syndrome
Rheumatological disorders,
   e.g. ankylosing spondylitis
   (aortic regurgitation)
Dyspnoea
Cyanosis
Jaundice
Cachexia

Hands
Radial pulses—right and left
Radiofemoral delay
Clubbing
Signs of infective endocarditis—
   splinter haemorrhages
Peripheral cyanosis
Xanthomata

Blood pressure

Face
Eyes
•   Sclerae—pallor, jaundice
•   Xanthelasma
•   Fundi—hypertensive changes
•   Malar flush (mitral stenosis,
    pulmonary stenosis)

Mouth
•   Cyanosis
•   Palate (high arched—Marfan's)
•   Dentition

Neck
•   Jugular venous pressure
•   Wave form (especially large v
    waves)
•   Carotids—pulse character

Figure 15.1　Examining the cardiovascular system.

Praecordium

Inspect
- Scars—whole chest, back
- Deformity
- Apex beat—position, character
- Abnormal pulsations

Palpate
- Apex beat—position, character
- Thrills
- Abnormal impulses

Auscultate

Heart sounds

Murmurs

Position patient
- Left lateral position
- Sitting forwards (forced expiratory apnoea)

NB: Palpate for thrills again after positioning

Dynamic auscultation
- Respiratory phases
- Valsalva

Back (sitting forwards)

Scars, deformity

Sacral oedema

Pleural effusion (percuss)

Left ventricular failure (auscultate)

Abdomen (lying flat—1 pillow only)

Palpate liver (pulsatile etc), spleen, aorta

Percuss for ascites (right heart failure)

Femoral arteries—palpate, auscultate

Legs

Peripheral pulses

Cyanosis, cold limbs, trophic changes, ulceration (peripheral vascular disease)

Oedema

Xanthomata

Calf tenderness

Clubbing of toes

Other

Urine analysis (infective endocarditis)

Fundi (endocarditis)

Temperature chart (endocarditis)

Figure 15.1, continued

or skin), **jaundice** (yellow discolouration of the skin and sclerae) and **cachexia** (generalised muscle wasting, which may be a result of cardiac failure).

3. Pick up the patient's right hand, then left.
   - Inspect the nails for **clubbing**.
   - Also look for the peripheral stigmata of infective endocarditis: **splinter haemorrhages** are common (and most often caused by trauma[2]).
   - Look quickly, but carefully, at each nail bed, otherwise it is easy to miss splinters.
   - Note any **tendon xanthomata** (hyperlipidaemia).
   - Time the pulse at the wrist for **rate** and **rhythm**.

---

2 Gardening is said to be the most common cause of splinter haemorrhages.

- Feel for **radiofemoral delay** (which occurs in coarctation of the aorta). Pulse character is best assessed at the carotids.

4. Measure the patient's **blood pressure** with the patient lying down. An initial high reading may necessitate retaking it after the patient has spent 5 or 10 minutes calming down. If there are symptoms of postural dizziness or loss of blood is suspected, the blood pressure should also be measured while the patient stands (to assess for postural hypotension).

5. Look at the patient's eyes again for **jaundice** (e.g. due to haemolysis caused by a prosthetic valve) or **conjunctival pallor** (anaemia) and eyelid **xanthelasma** (hyperlipidaemia). You may also notice the classic **mitral facies** (the bluish-red malar discolouration of mitral stenosis). Then inspect the mouth, using a torch, for the state of the **teeth** and **gums** (risk of endocarditis). Look at the tongue and lips for central **cyanosis**.

6. Assess the **jugular venous pressure** in the neck for height and character and the presence of **a waves** and **v waves**. Use the right internal jugular vein for this evaluation. This vein runs in the line between the angle of the jaw and the suprasternal notch. Look for a paradoxical rise of the JVP with inspiration (Kussmaul's sign). Feel each **carotid pulse** separately. Assess the pulse character.

7. **The praecordium.**
   - *Inspection.* Look for **scars**, **deformity**, the site of the apex beat and **visible pulsations**.
   - *Palpation.* Feel for the position of the **apex beat**. Count down the correct number of interspaces. The normal position is the fifth left intercostal space, 1 cm medial to the midclavicular line. The **character** of the apex beat should be noted (e.g. **pressure-loaded**, **volume-loaded**, **dyskinetic**). Feel for an apical thrill and, if it is present, time it (systolic or diastolic or both). Palpate with the heel of your hand for a left **parasternal impulse** (which indicates right ventricular enlargement or left atrial enlargement) and for thrills. Feel at the base of the heart for a **palpable pulmonary component** of the second heart sound (P2) and for aortic thrills.

- Percussion is unnecessary.
- *Auscultation.* Begin in the mitral area with first the bell and then the diaphragm. Listen for each component of the cardiac cycle separately.

8. Identify the **first** and **second heart sounds** and decide whether they are of normal intensity and whether the second heart sound is normally split. Listen for **extra heart sounds** and for **murmurs**. More than one abnormality may be present. Repeat the approach at the left sternal edge and then at the base of the heart (aortic and pulmonary areas). Time each part of the cycle with the carotid pulse. If a murmur is present, work out its timing and loudness and the effect of inspiration (vs expiration) on it.

9. Reposition the patient. First put the patient in the left lateral position. Again feel the apex beat for **character** (particularly tapping) and auscultate. Sit the patient up and palpate for **thrills** (with the patient in full expiration) at the left sternal edge and base. Then listen in those areas, particularly for aortic regurgitation.

10. Percuss the back of the patient's chest to exclude a **pleural effusion** (e.g. due to **left ventricular failure**) and auscultate for **inspiratory crackles** (left ventricular failure). If there is a radiofemoral delay, also listen for a coarctation murmur over the back. Feel for **sacral oedema**.

11. Next lay the patient flat and examine the abdomen properly for **hepatomegaly** (e.g. from **right ventricular failure**) and a **pulsatile liver** (**tricuspid regurgitation**). Feel for **splenomegaly** (e.g. endocarditis) and an **aortic aneurysm**. Palpate both femoral arteries and auscultate here for bruits.

12. Examine all the **peripheral pulses** (popliteal, dorsalis pedis and posterior tibial). Look for signs of **peripheral vascular disease**, peripheral **oedema**, clubbing of the toes, Achilles tendon **xanthomata** and stigmata of infective endocarditis. Look for varicose veins and leg ulceration.

13. Examine the urine for **haematuria** (e.g. endocarditis).

14. Examine the fundi for **hypertensive** changes.

15. Take the patient's **temperature** (e.g. endocarditis or other infection).

The respiratory system (see Fig 15.2)

1. Position the patient undressed to the waist and sitting over the side of the bed. Cover a woman's breasts with a towel or gown.

2. Inspect, while standing back, for **tachypnoea** at rest and any obvious asymmetry of movement. Count the **respiratory rate**. Look for the use of the **accessory muscles** of respiration. Cachexia should also be noted (e.g. malignancy). Look around the room for the all-important **sputum mug** and ask to see its contents (e.g. for haemoptysis).

3. Pick up the patient's hands.
   - Look for **clubbing**, peripheral **cyanosis**, **nicotine (tar) staining,** and **pallor** of the palmar creases suggesting anaemia.
   - Note any **wasting** of the small muscles of the hands (e.g. lung cancer involving the brachial plexus).
   - Palpate the **wrists** for **tenderness** (hypertrophic pulmonary osteoarthropathy).
   - Examine for a **flapping tremor** seen in carbon dioxide narcosis and liver failure.

4. Inspect the patient's face.
   - Look closely at the eyes for **constriction** of the **pupils** and ptosis (Horner's syndrome from an apical lung cancer).
   - Inspect the **tongue** for **central cyanosis**.

5. Palpate the position of the **trachea**. If the trachea is displaced, concentrate on the upper lobes for physical signs. Also note the presence of a **tracheal tug** (downward movement of the trachea with each inspiration, which indicates severe airflow obstruction). Ask the patient to speak (note **hoarseness**, which may be caused by recurrent laryngeal nerve palsy) and then cough, and note whether this is a loose cough, a dry cough or a bovine cough.

6. Examine the patient's **chest**. You may wish to examine the front first, or go to the back to start. The advantage of the latter is that there are often more signs there, unless the trachea is obviously displaced.

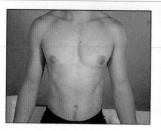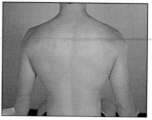

Position the patient sitting over the side of the bed.

General inspection
Type of cough
Use of supplementary oxygen
Rate and depth of respiration, and
   breathing pattern at rest
Accessory muscles of respiration
Sputum mug contents (blood, pus)

Hands
Clubbing
Cyanosis (peripheral)
Tar staining
Wasting, weakness—finger
   abduction and adduction (lung
   cancer involving the brachial
   plexus)
Wrist tenderness (hypertrophic
   pulmonary osteoarthropathy)
Pulse (tachycardia, pulsus paradoxus)
Flapping tremor (CO_2 narcosis)

Face
Eyes—Horner's syndrome (apical
   lung cancer), anaemia
Mouth—central cyanosis

Trachea
Voice—hoarseness (recurrent
   laryngeal nerve palsy)

Chest posteriorly
Inspect
- Shape of chest and spine
- Scars
- Prominent veins (determine
   direction of flow)
Palpate
- Cervical lymph nodes
- Expansion
- Vocal fremitus

Percuss
- Supraclavicular region

- Back of chest
- Axillae
Auscultate
- Breath sounds
- Adventitious sounds
- Vocal resonance

Chest anteriorly
Inspect
- Radiotherapy marks, other
   signs as noted above
Palpate
- Supraclavicular nodes
- Expansion
- Vocal fremitus
- Apex beat
Percuss
Auscultate
Pemberton's sign (superior vena
   cava obstruction)

Cardiovascular system (lying at 45°)
Jugular venous pressure (superior
   vena cava obstruction)
Cor pulmonale

Forced expiratory time

Other
Lower limbs—oedema, cyanosis
Temperature chart (infection)
Evidence of malignancy or pleural
   effusion: examine the breasts,
   liver, rectum, all lymph nodes

Figure 15.2 Examining the respiratory system.

7. If you start at the back, inspect the **spine**. Look for kyphoscoliosis and any signs of ankylosing spondylitis (which may cause decreased chest expansion and upper lobe fibrosis). Look for thoracotomy **scars**.

8. Palpate the **cervical nodes** from behind. Then examine for expansion—first **upper lobe expansion**, which is best assessed by looking over the patient's shoulders at clavicular movement during moderate respiration. The affected side will show a delay or decreased movement. Then examine **lower lobe expansion** by palpation. Note **asymmetry** and reduction of movement.

9. Ask the patient to bring the elbows together in the front to move the scapulae out of the way. Examine for **vocal fremitus**, then percuss the back of the chest.

10. Auscultate the back of the chest. Note **breath sounds** (whether **normal** or **bronchial**) and their intensity (**normal** or **reduced**). Listen for **adventitious sounds** (**crackles** and **wheezes**). Finally examine for **vocal resonance**. If a localised abnormality is found, try to determine the abnormal lobe.

11. Return to the front of the chest. Inspect again for chest deformity, **radiotherapy changes** and **scars**. Palpate the **supraclavicular nodes**. Then proceed with percussion and auscultation as before. Listen high up in the axillae, too. Before leaving the chest feel the axillary nodes and examine the breasts. Test for **Pemberton's sign**.

12. Lay the patient down at 45° and measure the **jugular venous pressure**. Then examine the **praecordium** for signs of pulmonary hypertension (**cor pulmonale**: a prominent parasternal impulse, palpable P2 and sometimes a right ventricular third or fourth heart sound and a murmur of tricuspid regurgitation).

13. Examine the **liver** (e.g. palpable because of ptosis or metastatic cancer, or pulsatile due to tricuspid regurgitation).

14. Take the patient's **temperature**.

The gastrointestinal system (see Fig 15.3)

1. Position the patient correctly with one pillow for the head and the abdomen completely exposed.

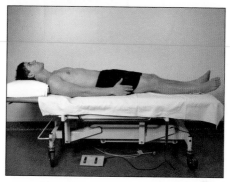

Position the patient lying flat on the bed with one pillow for the head and the abdomen completely exposed.

General inspection
Jaundice (liver disease)
Pigmentation (haemochromotosis, Whipple's disease)
Xanthomata (chronic cholestasis)
Mental state (encephalopathy)

Hands
Nails
- Clubbing
- Leuconychia
Palmar erythema
Dupuytren's contractures (alcohol)
Arthropathy
Hepatic flap

Arms
Spider naevi
Bruising
Wasting
Scratch marks (chronic cholestasis)

Face
Eyes
- Sclera: jaundice, anaemia, iritis
Parotids (alcohol)

Mouth
- Breath: fetor hepaticus
- Lips: stomatitis, leucoplakia, ulceration, localised pigmentation (Peutz–Jeghers syndrome), telangiectasia (hereditary haemorrhagic telangiectasia)
- Gums: gingivitis, bleeding, hypertrophy, pigmentation, monilia
- Tongue: atrophic glossitis, leucoplakia, ulceration

Cervical/axillary lymph nodes

Chest
Gynaecomastia
Spider naevi
Body hair loss

Abdomen
Inspect
- Scars
- Distension

Figure 15.3 Examining the gastrointestinal system. *continued*

- Prominent veins—determine direction of flow (caput medusae; inferior vena cava obstruction)
- Striae
- Bruising
- Pigmentation
- Localised masses
- Visible peristalsis

Palpate
- Superficial palpation—tenderness, rigidity, outline of any mass
- Deep palpation—organomegaly (liver, spleen, kidney), abnormal masses

Roll on to right side and palpate (spleen)

Percuss
- Viscera outline
- Ascites—shifting dullness

Auscultate
- Bowel sounds
- Bruits, hums
- Rubs

Groin
Genitalia
Lymph nodes
Hernial orifices (standing up)

Legs
Bruising
Oedema
Neurological signs (alcohol)

Other
Rectal examination—inspect (fistulae, tags, blood, mucus), palpate (masses)
Urine analysis (bile)
Cardiovascular system (jugular venous pressure, signs of right heart failure if hepatomegaly)
Temperature chart (infection)

Figure 15.3, continued

2. Look, while standing back, at the general appearance and for obvious signs of chronic liver disease.
3. Pick up the patient's hands.
   - Ask the patient to extend his or her arms and hands and look for **asterixis**.
   - Look also at the nails for **clubbing** and for **liver (white) nails**.
   - Note the presence of **palmar erythema** or **Dupuytren's contractures**.
4. Look at the arms for **bruising**, **scratch marks**, **spider naevi** and proximal muscle wasting.
5. Go to the face.
   - Note any scleral changes (e.g. **jaundice**, **anaemia**) or **iritis**.
   - Feel for parotid enlargement, then inspect the mouth with a torch and spatula for **angular stomatitis**.
   - Smell the breath for **fetor hepaticus**.
6. Look at the chest for **spider naevi**, and in men for **gynaecomastia** and loss of body hair.

7. Inspect the abdomen from the side, squatting to the patient's level. Large masses may be visible. Ask the patient to take slow deep breaths and look for the outlines of the liver, spleen and gall bladder. If distended, note whether this is central, peripheral or in one flank.

8. Palpate lightly in each region for **masses**, having asked first whether any area is particularly tender. This will avoid causing pain and may provide a clue to sites of possible pathology. Next palpate more deeply in each region, then feel specifically for **hepatomegaly** and **splenomegaly**. If there is hepatomegaly, confirm this with percussion and estimate the span (normal <13 cm). Repeat this procedure for splenomegaly. Always roll the patient onto the right side and palpate again if the spleen is not felt at first. Attempt now to feel the kidneys bimanually.

9. Percuss for **ascites**. If the abdomen is resonant right out to the flanks, do not roll the patient over. Otherwise, test for **shifting dullness**.

10. By auscultation note the presence of **bowel sounds**. Listen also for **bruits**, **hums** and **rubs**. Always auscultate over the liver, spleen or kidneys if these are enlarged or palpable, or over any palpable **mass**.

11. Examine the groin. Palpate for **inguinal lymphadenopathy**. Examine for **hernias** by asking the patient to stand and then cough. The **testes** in men must be palpated.

12. Now look at the legs for **oedema** and **bruising**. Neurological examination of the legs may be indicated if there are signs of chronic liver disease (e.g. from alcohol abuse).

13. If the liver is **enlarged** or cirrhosis is suspected, the patient should be sat up to 45° and the jugular venous pressure estimated (to exclude right heart failure as a cause of liver disease).

14. While the patient is sitting up, palpate in the **supraclavicular fossae** for lymph nodes and feel over the lower back for **sacral oedema**. If ascites is present, it is necessary to examine the chest for pleural effusions. If malignant disease is suspected, examine all the lymph node groups, the breasts and the lungs.

15. A **rectal examination** should be performed and specimens of the patient's vomitus or faeces should be inspected, if available.

The genitourinary system (see Fig 15.4)

1. Lay the patient flat on the bed while making the usual general inspection. Note particularly the patient's mental state and whether the patient has a sallow complexion, the state of **hydration** and whether the patient is **hiccupping** or **hyperventilating** (possible signs of renal failure).

2. Pick up the patient's hands and look at the nails for **leuconychia** or white transverse lines that may occur in hypoalbuminaemia (e.g. nephrotic syndrome).

3. Examine the patient's wrists and arms for vascular access sites.
   - Assess the patency of an **arteriovenous fistula** by palpating for a thrill. Get the patient to hold out his or her hands and look for **asterixis**.
   - Then inspect the patient's arms for **subcutaneous nodules** (e.g. calcium phosphate deposits), bruising, pigmentation and scratch marks (chronic kidney disease).

4. Go on to the face.
   - Begin by examining the eyes for **anaemia** (chronic kidney disease).
   - Examine the mouth for **dryness** (dehydration) or **fetor**.
   - Note the presence of any vasculitic rash on the face. Note any neck scars (e.g. parathyroid surgery).

5. Lay the patient flat and examine the abdomen.
   - Look for **scars** indicating peritoneal dialysis or operations including a **renal transplant**.
   - Then examine the liver and spleen (enlargement may occur in polycystic disease). Palpate for **enlarged kidneys by ballottement**.
   - Feel for the presence of an **abdominal aortic aneurysm**. Percuss over the bladder to detect enlargement.
   - Listen for aortic and renal bruits.

6. Sit the patient up and palpate the back for tenderness and sacral oedema.

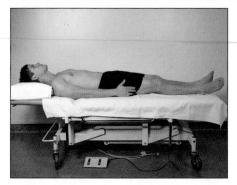

General inspection
Mental state
Hyperventilation (acidosis), hiccups
Hydration
Subcutaneous nodules (calcium
  phosphate deposits)

Hands
Nails—leuconychia; white transverse
  lines; single white band; distal nail
  brown, proximal nail white or pink
  (half-and-half nails)

Arms
Bruising
Pigmentation
Scratch marks
Myopathy

Face
Eyes—anaemia, jaundice, band
  keratopathy
Mouth—dryness, ulcers, fetor
Rash (vasculitis)

Abdomen
Scars—dialysis, operations
Kidneys—transplant kidney
Bladder
Liver
Lymph nodes
Ascites
Rectal examination (prostatomegaly)

Back
Tenderness
Oedema

Chest
Heart—pericarditis, failure
Lungs—infection, pulmonary
  oedema

Legs
Oedema—nephrotic syndrome,
  cardiac failure
Bruising
Pigmentation
Scratch marks
Neuropathy
Vascular access

Urine analysis
Specific gravity, pH
Glucose—diabetes mellitus
Blood—nephritis, infection, stone
Protein—nephritis, nephrotic
  syndrome

Other
Blood pressure—lying and standing
Fundoscopy—hypertensive and
  diabetic changes

Figure 15.4 Examining the genitourinary system.

7. Look at the **jugular venous pressure** with the patient at 45°. Examine the heart for signs of pericarditis, pericardial effusion or cardiac failure and the lungs for pulmonary oedema.

8. Lay the patient down again.
   - Look at the legs for **oedema** (due to the **nephrotic syndrome** or **cardiac failure**), bruising, pigmentation, scratch marks or the presence of gout.
   - Examine for **peripheral neuropathy** (decreased sensation, loss of reflexes in chronic renal failure).

9. Measure the **blood pressure** with the patient lying down and then standing (for **orthostatic** [postural] **hypotension**) and perform **fundoscopy** to look for hypertensive or diabetic changes.

10. Perform a rectal examination, if indicated, to feel for **prostatomegaly**.

11. Finally, perform **urinalysis**, testing for specific gravity, pH, glucose, blood, protein and leucocytes.

The haematological system (see Fig 15.5)

1. Position the patient as for a gastrointestinal examination and make sure he or she is fully undressed.

2. Look for **bruising**, **pigmentation**, **cyanosis**, **jaundice** and **scratch marks** (suggesting pruritis due to myelo-proliferative disease or lymphoma). Look for frontal bossing and note the racial origin of the patient (e.g. in thalassaemia).

3. Pick up the patient's hands.
   - Look at the **nails** for **koilonychia** (spoon-shaped nails—iron deficiency) and the changes of **vasculitis**.
   - Pale palmar creases may indicate **anaemia**.
   - Evidence of **arthropathy** may be important (e.g. **rheumatoid arthritis** and **Felty's syndrome**, recurrent **haemarthroses** in bleeding disorders, secondary **gout** in myeloproliferative disorders).

4. Examine the **epitrochlear** nodes.

5. Note any bruising on the arms. Remember, **petechiae** are pinhead haemorrhages, while **ecchymoses** are larger bruises. Palpable purpura indicates a vasculitis.

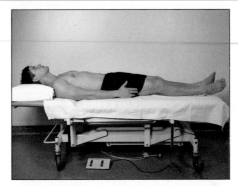

Position the patient lying flat on the bed with one pillow for the head.

General inspection
Bruising (thrombocytopenia, scurvy, haemophilia)
- Petechia (pinhead bleeding)
- Ecchymoses (large bruises)

Pigmentation (lymphoma)
Rashes and infiltrative lesions (lymphoma)
Ulceration (neutropenia)
Cyanosis (polycythaemia)
Plethora (polycythaemia)
Jaundice (haemolysis)
Scratch marks (myeloproliferative diseases, lymphoma)
Racial origin
Pallor (anaemia)

Hands
Nails—koilonychia
Palmar crease pallor (anaemia)
Arthropathy (haemophilia, secondary gout, drug treatment)

Epitrochlear nodes

Axillary nodes

Face
Sclera—jaundice, pallor, conjunctival suffusion (polycythaemia)
Mouth—gum hypertrophy (monocytic leukaemia), ulceration, infection, haemorrhage (marrow aplasia); atrophic glossitis, angular stomatitis (iron, vitamin deficiencies)

Cervical nodes (sitting up)
Palpate from behind

Bony tenderness
Spine
Sternum
Clavicles
Shoulders

Abdomen (lying flat) and genitalia
Organomegaly (spleen, liver)
Inguinal nodes

Legs
Vasculitis (Henoch-Schönlein purpura—buttocks, thighs)
Bruising
Pigmentation
Ulceration (e.g. haemo-globinopathies)
Neurological signs (subacute combined degeneration in vitamin B_{12} deficiency, peripheral neuropathy)

Other
Fundi (haemorrhages, infection)
Temperature chart (infection)
Urine analysis (haematuria, bile)
Rectal and pelvic examination (blood loss)

Figure 15.5 Examining the haematological system.

6. Go to the axillae and palpate the **axillary** nodes. There are five main areas:
   - central
   - lateral (above and lateral)
   - pectoral (most medial)
   - infraclavicular (apical)
   - subscapular (most inferior).
7. Look at the face. Inspect the eyes, note jaundice, pallor or haemorrhage of the sclerae, and the injected sclerae of **polycythaemia**.
8. Examine the mouth.
   - Note gum **hypertrophy** (e.g. from acute monocytic leukaemia or scurvy), ulceration, infection, haemorrhage, **atrophic glossitis** (e.g. from iron deficiency, or vitamin B_{12} or folate deficiency) and angular stomatitis.
   - Look for tonsillar and adenoid enlargement (e.g. leukaemia).
9. Sit the patient up.
   - Examine the **cervical nodes** from behind: submental, submandibular, jugular chain, posterior triangle, postauricular, preauricular and occipital.
   - Then feel the **supraclavicular area** from the front.
10. Tap the **spine** with your fist for **bony tenderness** (which may be caused by an enlarging marrow—e.g. in myeloma or carcinoma). Press gently on the sternum, clavicles and shoulders for bony tenderness.
11. Lay the patient flat again.
    - Examine the abdomen. Note any splenomegaly, hepatomegaly or para-aortic nodes (rarely palpable).
    - Examine the inguinal lymph nodes.
    - Don't forget to palpate the testes in men.
    - Consider performing a rectal (and pelvic examination) for evidence of bleeding.
    - Spring the hips for pelvic tenderness.
12. Examine the legs.
    - Note particularly **leg ulcers** (e.g. due to haemolytic anaemia, thalassaemia, Felty's syndrome and polycythaemia).
    - Examine the legs from a **neurological** aspect, for peripheral neuropathy (e.g. vitamin B_{12} deficiency,

which also causes posterior column loss and upper motor neuron signs).

13. Examine the **fundi**, look at the **temperature** chart and test the **urine**.

The nervous system (see Fig 15.6)

1. **Handedness**, **orientation** and **speech**.
   - Ask the patient whether he or she is right- or left-handed.
   - As a screening assessment, ask the patient to state his or her name, the present location and the date.
   - Next ask the patient to name an object pointed at and then ask the patient to point to a named object in the room (to test for dysphasia).

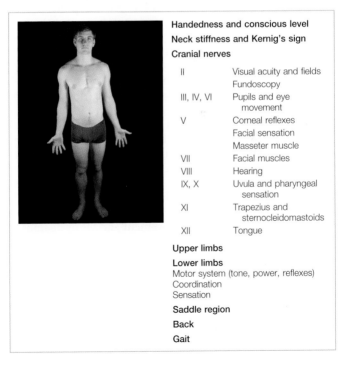

Handedness and conscious level

Neck stiffness and Kernig's sign

Cranial nerves

II	Visual acuity and fields
	Fundoscopy
III, IV, VI	Pupils and eye movement
V	Corneal reflexes
	Facial sensation
	Masseter muscle
VII	Facial muscles
VIII	Hearing
IX, X	Uvula and pharyngeal sensation
XI	Trapezius and sternocleidomastoids
XII	Tongue

Upper limbs

Lower limbs
Motor system (tone, power, reflexes)
Coordination
Sensation

Saddle region

Back

Gait

Figure 15.6   Examining the nervous system.

- Ask the patient to say 'British constitution' (to test for dysarthria).

2. **Neck stiffness and Kernig's sign.** If the symptom onset is acute, look for these signs of meningism.

3. **Cranial nerves.** The patient should be sat over the edge of the bed, if possible.
   - Begin with a general inspection of the head and neck, looking for craniotomy scars, neurofibromas, facial asymmetry, ptosis, proptosis, skew deviation of the eyes or pupil inequality.
   - **The second nerve.**
     - Test visual acuity with the patient wearing his or her spectacles. Test each eye separately, while the other is covered with a small card.
     - Examine the visual fields by confrontation, using a hatpin. If visual acuity is very poor, map the fields using your fingers.
     - Look into the fundi.
   - **The third, fourth and sixth nerves.**
     - Look at the pupils, noting the shape, relative sizes and any associated **ptosis**. Use a pocket torch and shine the light from the side to gauge the reaction of the pupils to light.
     - Assess both the **direct** and **consensual** responses. Test **accommodation** by asking the patient to look into the distance and then at the hatpin placed about 20 cm from the nose.
     - Assess **eye movements** with both eyes first, getting the patient to follow the pin in each direction.
     - Ask about **diplopia**.
     - Look for **failure of movement** and for **nystagmus**.
   - **The fifth nerve.**
     - Test the **corneal reflexes** gently and ask the patient whether the touch of cottonwool on the cornea can be felt. The sensory component of this reflex is the fifth nerve and the motor component is the seventh nerve.
     - Test **facial sensation** in the three divisions: **ophthalmic**, **maxillary** and **mandibular**. Test **pain** sensation with a new pin and map any area of sensory loss from dull to sharp. Test light touch as

well so that **sensory dissociation** can be detected, if present.

- Examine the motor division of the fifth nerve by asking the patient to **clench the teeth** while you feel the masseter muscles.
- Then get the patient to open his or her mouth while you attempt to force it closed. A unilateral lesion causes the **jaw to deviate** towards the weak (affected) side.
- Test the **jaw jerk**. With the patient's mouth open, tap with a tendon hammer one of your own fingers placed on the patient's chin. Brisk closure of the mouth occurs in an upper motor neuron lesion.

- **The seventh nerve.** Test the muscles of facial expression.
    - Ask the patient to look up and **wrinkle the forehead**. Look for loss of wrinkling and feel the muscle strength by pushing down on each side.
    - Next ask the patient to **shut his or her eyes** tightly and compare the two sides.
    - Ask the patient to **grin** so that you can compare the nasolabial grooves.
- **The eighth nerve.**
    - Whisper a number 60 cm away from each of the patient's ears.
    - Perform **Rinné's** and **Weber's** tests with a 256-Hz tuning fork if there is deafness.
    - Examine the external auditory canals and the eardrums, if this is indicated.
- **The ninth and tenth nerves.**
    - Look at the palate and note any **uvular** displacement.
    - Ask the patient to say 'ah' and look for symmetrical movement of the soft palate (tenth).
    - Test gently for **pharyngeal sensation** (the ninth nerve is the sensory component and the tenth nerve the motor component if a gag reflex occurs).
    - Ask the patient to speak to assess hoarseness, and to cough and swallow.

- **The eleventh nerve.**
  - Ask the patient to shrug his or her shoulders, and feel the **trapezius** while pushing the shoulders down.
  - Then ask the patient to turn his or her head against resistance, and also feel the bulk of the **sternocleidomastoid**.
- **The twelfth nerve.**
  - While examining the patient's mouth, inspect the tongue for wasting and fasciculation.
  - Next ask the patient to protrude the tongue. Unilateral paralysis results in **deviation of the tongue** towards the paralysed side.
- Then examine the skull and auscultate for carotid bruits.

4. **Upper limbs**. Ask the patient to sit over the side of the bed facing you.
   - Examine the **motor system** systematically every time. Inspect first for wasting and fasciculations.
   - Ask the patient to hold out both hands with the arms extended and to close the eyes (see Fig 15.7). Look for **drifting** of one or both arms (caused by an upper motor neuron weakness, a cerebellar lesion or posterior column loss).

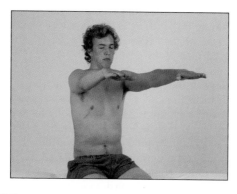

Figure 15.7   Testing for arm drift.

- Also note any **tremor** or **pseudoathetosis** due to proprioceptive loss. Feel the **muscle bulk** and note any muscle tenderness.
- Test **tone** at the wrists and elbows by passively moving the joints at varying velocities.
- Assess **power** at the shoulders, elbows, wrists and fingers.
- If indicated, test for an ulnar nerve lesion (Froment's sign) and a median nerve lesion (pen-touching test).
- Examine the **reflexes**: biceps (C5, C6), triceps (C7, C8), brachioradialis (C5, C6) and finger jerks (C8).
- Assess **coordination** with finger–nose testing and look for dysdiadochokinesis and rebound.
- Examine the **sensory system** after motor testing because this can be time-consuming. First test the **spinothalamic pathway** (pain). Start proximally and test each dermatome.
- Next test the **posterior column** pathway. Use a 128-Hz tuning fork to assess **vibration** sense. Place the vibrating fork on a distal interphalangeal joint initially.
- Examine **proprioception** with the distal interphalangeal joint of the index finger.
- Test **light touch** with cottonwool. Touch the skin lightly (do not stroke) in each dermatome.
- Feel for thickened nerves—the ulnar at the elbow, and the median and radial at the wrist—and feel the axillae if there is evidence of a proximal lesion. Note any scars, and finally examine the neck, if relevant.

5. **Lower limbs**.
   - Test the **stance** and **gait** first, if possible (see Fig 15.8).
     - Ask the patient to walk normally for a few metres and then turn around quickly and walk back.
     - Then ask the patient to walk heel-to-toe to exclude a mid-line cerebellar lesion.
     - Ask the patient to walk on the toes (an S1 lesion will make this impossible) and then on the heels (an L4 or L5 lesion causing footdrop will make this impossible).
     - Look for shuffling (Parkinson's disease), hemiplegia (the foot is swung in an arc and remains plantarflexed) or a wide-based gait (cerebellar disease).

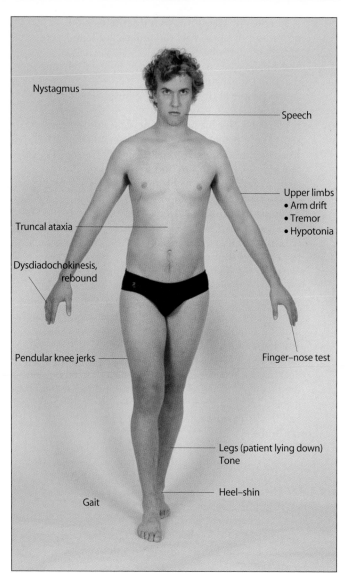

Nystagmus

Speech

Upper limbs
• Arm drift
• Tremor
• Hypotonia

Truncal ataxia

Dysdiadochokinesis,
rebound

Pendular knee jerks

Finger–nose test

Legs (patient lying down)
Tone

Heel–shin

Gait

Figure 15.8 Signs of cerebellar disease.

- Ask the patient to lie on the bed with his or her legs entirely exposed.
  - Note any fasciculations.
  - Feel the muscle bulk of the quadriceps and run your hand up each shin, feeling for wasting of the anterior tibial muscles.
- Test **tone** at the knees and ankles. Test **clonus** at the knee and ankle.
- Assess **power** at the hips, knees and ankles.
- Elicit the **reflexes**: knee (L3, L4), ankle (S1, S2) and plantar response (L5, S1, S2).
- Test **coordination** with the heel–shin test, toe–finger test and tapping of the feet.
- Examine the **sensory system** as for the upper limbs: pin-prick, then vibration and proprioception (beginning with the big toe), and then light touch. If there is sensory loss involving the whole leg or legs, attempt to establish a sensory level on the trunk and abdomen. Examine **sensation in the saddle region** and test the **anal reflex** (S2, S3, S4).
- Look for deformity, scars and neurofibromas on the patient's back. Palpate for tenderness over the vertebral bodies and auscultate for bruits. Perform the **straight leg raising test**.

16 Writing and presenting the history and physical examination

Study sickness while you are well.

Thomas Fuller (1608–1661)

Writing up the history and physical examination

The written entries in a patient's notes are an important legal document. The notes may be used for reference throughout the patient's admission and during any future admissions to hospital. The initial admitting notes are usually the most comprehensive. A system for recording these is outlined below. The exact format, however, will be different for different types of admission. The routine admission of a young person for a minor surgical procedure under local anaesthetic will be much less detailed than the admission of an elderly patient with a complicated medical problem.

Further entries to the notes usually record ward rounds and decisions by the treating team about investigations and treatment. If a patient becomes acutely ill on the ward, a record must be made of the details of the problem, the examination findings, the proposed investigations and their results, and the advice of the senior staff who have been consulted. The entry must be updated frequently if the patient's condition changes.

The history

PERSONAL INFORMATION

Record the patient's name, gender and date of birth. Write down the date and time of the examination.

PRESENTING (PRINCIPAL) SYMPTOMS (PS)

A short sentence identifies the major presenting complaints and their duration; it is very helpful to quote the patient's own words.

HISTORY OF PRESENT ILLNESS (HPI)

Do not record every detail; rather, prepare short prose paragraphs or use dot points telling the story of the illness in chronological order (from the past to the present time). Describe the characteristics of each symptom. Note the reason for the patient's presentation at this time. Describe any current treatment (and the proposed diagnosis if known). Also describe any past medical problems that are related to the current symptoms. Include the relevant positive and negative findings on the systems review here.

If there are many seemingly unrelated problems, summarise these in an introductory paragraph and present the history of each problem in a separate paragraph. Record your impression of the reliability of the historian and, if the patient was unable to give the history, describe who the source was.

MEDICATIONS

List the patient's current medications (including any over-the-counter medications) and doses, the indications for their use (if known) and any side effects. The medication list may give a clue to chronic medical conditions the patient may have neglected to mention (e.g. use of anti-hypertensive drugs).

PAST HISTORY (PH)

List in chronological order past medical problems and surgical operations, and past medication use, if relevant. Record any history of allergy (particularly drug allergy). A history of blood transfusions should be noted.

SOCIAL HISTORY (SH)

Describe as a minimum the patient's occupation, marital status and recent travel. Smoking habits, alcohol use, analgesic use and other non-medical drug use should also be described.

FAMILY HISTORY (FH)

Describe causes of mortality or relevant morbidity in the patient's first-degree relatives and, if indicated, draw a family tree.

SYSTEMS REVIEW (SR)

All directly relevant information should be incorporated into the HPI or PH.

The physical examination (PE)

Under each of the major systems, list the relevant positives and negatives using brief statements (see Fig 16.1). Begin with the system most relevant to the presenting symptoms.

Provisional diagnosis, problem list and plans

Using a sentence or two, summarise the most important findings and then give a provisional diagnosis (PD) and list the differential diagnosis (DD). List all the active problems that require management. Outline the diagnostic tests and therapy planned for each problem. Sign your name and then print your name and position underneath.

Personal details

Name: Mr W Witheridge
Age: 72
Occupation: Retired botanist

Presenting symptoms

3 weeks of progressive exertional dyspnoea with 2 days of dyspnoea at rest.

History of present illness

Two nights of severe orthopnoea; unable to sleep except briefly while sitting in a chair.
Mild exertional shortness of breath for nearly 10 years.
Unable to walk 50 metres on the flat.
No associated chest tightness or pain.
No wheeze or cough.
No fever.
No recent change in medications.
No asthma or known lung disease. No other relevant positive symptoms on systems review.

Past cardiac history

Previous myocardial infarction 5 years ago, treated with thrombolytic drugs. No known valvular heart disease or history of rheumatic fever. Smoked 25 cigarettes a day until the time of his infarct—30 packet years.

Risk factors for heart disease

Total cholesterol 6.7 mmol/L, a family history of ischaemic heart disease—his 55-year-old brother had hypertension for 30 years—inadequate control. Salt intake high, drinks 3-4 litres of fluid a day. Alcohol—25 g a week. There is no history of diabetes mellitus. Only occasional non-steroidal anti-inflammatory drugs.

Other symptoms

10 years of nocturia three times per night. He denies other urinary tract symptoms.

Current medications

Aspirin, 100 mg daily; metoprolol (a beta-blocker), 100 mg twice a day. No use of over-the-counter medications.

Past history

Gastric ulceration 3 years ago—successfully treated with a 14-day course of antibiotics and a proton pump inhibitor; no recurrence of symptoms. Appendectomy and tonsillectomy in his youth.

Figure 16.1 An example of a medical history.

He has no drug allergies that he knows of and has never required a blood transfusion.

Social history

Lives in retirement with his wife, who is well.
Interests: gardening, history of medicinal plants. No other hobbies. No pets.
No recent overseas travel.

Family history

His father died of a myocardial infarct at age 64 years and his mother died of colon cancer at age 84 years. Both sons (42 and 39 years) are alive and well. No other relevant family history.

Physical examination

Breathless and uncomfortable at rest. Temperature 37°C.
Respiratory rate—24 breaths per minute.

Cardiovascular

No cyanosis. No clubbing. No splinter haemorrhages.
Pulse rate 90 beats per minute and regular.
Blood pressure 180/110 mmHg, lying and standing.
JVP not elevated.
Apex beat 2 cm displaced, dyskinetic.
Heart sounds (HS): S1 and S2 present and normal; S3 present.
Pansystolic murmur grade 3/6 maximum at the apex consistent with mitral regurgitation.

Chest

Trachea in the mid-line.
Expansion normal right and left.
Normal percussion note bilaterally.
Bilateral medium basal mid-inspiratory crackles and occasional expiratory wheeze over the right and left lung fields. No areas of bronchial breathing.

Abdomen

Well-healed appendix scar present.
Abdomen soft, no tenderness.
Liver not palpable, no other masses (spleen, kidneys).
No ascites.
Normal bowel sounds.
Rectal examination deferred (the patient was too unwell at the time of admission).

Figure 16.1, continued

Legs

No calf tenderness.
No peripheral oedema.
Peripheral pulses present and equal.
No visible varicose veins.

Central nervous system (CNS)

Alert and orientated.
No neck stiffness.

Cranial nerves (assessed after initial treatment)

II—acuity and fields normal; fundi normal.
III, IV and VI—pupils equal, circular and concentric—react normally to light and accommodation; eye movements normal; no nystagmus.
V—sensation and motor function normal.
VII—muscles of facial expression normal.
VIII—hearing normal.
IX, X—no uvular displacement.
XI—normal power.
XII—no fasciculation or displacement of tongue.

Upper limbs

No wasting, fasciculations, tremor.
Tone normal.
Power normal (shoulders, elbows, wrists, fingers).
Reflexes normal and symmetrical.[1]

	Right	Left
Biceps	++	++
Triceps	++	++
Brachioradialis	++	++

Coordination normal.
Sensation—pain, proprioception normal.

Figure 16.1, continued

---

1 The reflexes can be recorded as:

O (absent)
+ (reduced)
++ (normal)
+++ (increased)
++++ (exaggerated with clonus)

Lower limbs
Gait normal.
No wasting.
Tone normal; no clonus.
Power normal (hips, knees, ankles).
Reflexes normal and symmetrical.

	Right	*Left*
Knee	++	++
Ankle	++	++
Plantars	↓	↓ (normal)

Coordination normal.
Sensation—pain, proprioception normal.

Provisional diagnosis: left ventricular failure secondary to ischaemic heart disease.
Differential diagnosis: angina, pulmonary embolus, chronic obstructive pulmonary disease.
Investigations:
*   Electrocardiogram*
*   Chest X-ray*
*   Full blood count*
*   Electrolytes, creatinine, liver function tests*
*   Echocardiogram*

Comment
The aetiology of his cardiac failure is most likely to be ischaemic heart disease (previous infarct) or hypertensive. He has signs of mitral regurgitation, which may be secondary to cardiac failure or, less likely, the cause. There is no known history of chronic lung disease, although he has been a chronic smoker. The history and examination are not very suggestive of pulmonary embolism.

Figure 16.1, continued

Presenting the history and physical examination

It is not enough to take a history, examine a patient and make a diagnosis. You must also be able to pass this information on by means of written notes and case presentations to colleagues and others involved in the patient's care.

PRESENTING IN THE LONG CASE EXAM

The presentation of a patient's history and physical examination to examiners (a long case exam) is a very formal exercise. An effective approach is to begin by giving the examiners information about the patient's age and sex, and then to explain whether it is a diagnostic problem or a treatment problem, or both. For example, you might say: 'I am presenting Mrs X, a 75-year-old woman with a diagnostic and management problem of the sudden onset of left-sided weakness.' This lets the examiners know that you have thought about the problem and are not just presenting a series of facts.

The presentation should continue, starting with more detail about the presenting symptoms. It is important not to bore the examiners with long lists of irrelevant negative physical examination findings, but to have this information available if asked for it. At the end of your presentation you should present a differential diagnosis (in order of likelihood) and a proposed plan of investigation and treatment (management).

PRESENTING TO A CONSULTANT

The long case format is not the best way to present a patient's details to a senior colleague, especially in the middle of the night. There are three reasons for contacting a consultant about a new patient:

1. A polite call to let the consultant know about a patient who is stable. Some consultants want to know about new patients at any time, while others are happy to be told when it is convenient (e.g. after grand rounds are over, at a reasonable hour of the morning or when a series of routine admissions has been saved up).
2. A call to seek advice and discuss the proposed management of a patient who has complications.
3. A call to ask the consultant to come in to see the patient or to perform a procedure.

The reason for the call should be given at the start of the conversation. Consultants are rarely interested in hearing a long list of irrelevant negative findings. The appropriate course is to give a brief history of the presenting problem and objective findings, followed by a differential diagnosis and management plan. Then stop talking to allow for discussion or approval of the plan.

PRESENTING AT A HANDOVER MEETING

Here the patient is being presented to colleagues who will be taking over the management of the patient. These meetings vary in formality. It is essential that patients who are unwell or have unresolved problems be discussed in the greatest detail. The team taking over care of the patient needs to know where the patient is, some biographical details about the patient, and briefly the presenting clinical features and provisional diagnosis.

Investigations that are available must be outlined and those that have been ordered but are not yet available identified so that these results are not missed. A sick patient may need urgent and frequent review by the new team.

If consultants or senior registrars are present, their advice should be sought about more difficult patients.

Often a particular patient is chosen for more detailed discussion as a teaching exercise. This patient's history and examination findings may have to be outlined in relatively more detail, but not to the point of a long case presentation.

T&O'C examination hint box

Here are some common abbreviations used in patients' notes (but these do vary so be careful—it is best to spell out most terms in the notes, to avoid miscommunication!).

Abd.	Abdomen
AJ	Ankle jerk
AR	Aortic regurgitation
AS	Aortic stenosis
ASD	Atrial septal defect
BS	Breath sounds or bowel sounds
BP	Blood pressure
CNS	Central nervous system
CP	Chest pain
Cx	Circumflex (coronary artery)
CXR	Chest X-ray
dp	Dorsalis pedis (pulse)
HPI	History of the presenting illness

HS	Heart sounds
JVP	Jugular venous pulse/pressure
KJ	Knee jerk
LAD	Left anterior descending (coronary artery)
LMO	Local medical officer
MR	Mitral regurgitation
MS	Mitral stenosis or multiple sclerosis
O/E	On examination
PDA	Patent ductus arteriosus
PCCRLA	Pupils concentric, central, reacting to light and accommodation
Plantars	Plantar reflexes
PH	Past history
PND	Paroxysmal nocturnal dyspnoea
PS	Presenting symptoms
PPs	Peripheral pulses
PR	Per rectal (examination)
Pt	Posterior tibial (artery)
Rx	Medications or treatment
SOBOE	Short of breath on exertion
Sx	Surgery or surgical history
S3, S4	Third heart sound, fourth heart sound
Tx	Thyrotoxicosis or transplant
VSD	Ventricular septal defect
°	Absent e.g. BS° bowel sounds absent
$\sqrt{}$	Present e.g. HS$\sqrt{}^2$ heart sounds present
+++	Brisk reflex

---

2 Suggests limited auscultation skills.

List of OSCEs

Final remarks

He has been a doctor a year now and has had two patients, no, three, I think—yes, it was three; I attended their funerals.

Samuel Clemens (Mark Twain) (1835–1910)

Medical education is not completed at the Medical school; it is only begun.

William H Welch (1850–1934)

You should now be well on your way in your journey towards acquiring the vital clinical skills of history taking and physical examination. Despite the increasing acceleration of technological innovation in the medical field, these are the skills that you will utilise throughout your medical career. Of course, the journey will never end, because learning and relearning these skills is a lifelong occupation.

Good luck!

Index

Page numbers followed by '*f*' indicate figures, '*t*' indicate tables and '*b*' indicate boxes.